Cutting-Edge Trauma and Emergency Care

Editors

MAUREEN MCCUNN
MOHAMMED IQBAL AHMED
CATHERINE M. KUZA

ANESTHESIOLOGY CLINICS

www.anesthesiology.theclinics.com

Consulting Editor
LEE A. FLEISHER

March 2019 • Volume 37 • Number 1

ELSEVIER

1600 John F. Kennedy Boulevard • Suite 1800 • Philadelphia, Pennsylvania, 19103-2899

http://www.theclinics.com

ANESTHESIOLOGY CLINICS Volume 37, Number 1
March 2019 ISSN 1932-2275, ISBN-13: 978-0-323-67813-1

Editor: Colleen Dietzler
Developmental Editor: Kristen Helm

Anesthesiology Clinics (ISSN 1932-2275) is published quarterly by Elsevier Inc., 360 Park Avenue South, New York, NY 10010-1710. Months of issue are March, June, September, and December. Periodicals postage paid at New York, NY and at additional mailing offices. Subscription prices are $100.00 per year (US student/resident), $360.00 per year (US individuals), $446.00 per year (Canadian individuals), $693.00 per year (US institutions), $876.00 per year (Canadian institutions), $225.00 per year (Canadian and foreign student/resident), $469.00 per year (foreign individuals), and $876.00 per year (foreign institutions). To receive student and resident rate, orders must be accompanied by name of affiliated institution, date of term, and the *signature* of program/residency coordinator on institutions letterhead. Orders will be billed at individual rate until proof of status is received. Foreign air speed delivery is included in all *Clinics'* subscription prices. All prices are subject to change without notice. POSTMASTER: Send address changes to *Anesthesiology Clinics,* Elsevier Health Sciences Division, Subscription Customer Service, 3251 Riverport Lane, Maryland Heights, MO 63043. Customer Service (orders, claims, online, change of address): Elsevier Health Sciences Division, Subscription Customer Service, 3251 Riverport Lane, Maryland Heights, MO 63043. **Tel:1-800-654-2452 (U.S. and Canada); 314-447-8871 (outside U.S. and Canada). Fax: 314-447-8029. E-mail: journalscustomerservice-usa@elsevier.com (for print support); journalsonlinesupport-usa@elsevier.com (for online support).**

Reprints. For copies of 100 or more of articles in this publication, please contact the Commercial Reprints Department, Elsevier Inc., 360 Park Avenue South, New York, NY 10010-1710. Tel.: 212-633-3874; Fax: 212-633-3820; E-mail: reprints@elsevier.com.

Anesthesiology Clinics, is also published in Spanish by McGraw-Hill Inter-americana Editores S. A., P.O. Box 5-237, 06500 Mexico D. F., Mexico.

Anesthesiology Clinics, is covered in *MEDLINE/PubMed (Index Medicus), Current Contents/Clinical Medicine, Excerpta Medica, ISI/BIOMED,* and *Chemical Abstracts.*

Contributors

CONSULTING EDITOR

LEE A. FLEISHER, MD, FACC, FAHA
Robert D. Dripps Professor and Chair of Anesthesiology and Critical Care, Professor of Medicine, Perelman School of Medicine, University of Pennsylvania, Philadelphia, Pennsylvania, USA

EDITORS

MAUREEN MCCUNN, MD, MIPP, FCCM, FASA
Professor, Department of Anesthesiology, University of Maryland School of Medicine, Division of Trauma Anesthesiology, R Adams Cowley Shock Trauma Center, Board of Directors, Trauma Anesthesiology Society, Chair, American Society of Anesthesiologists Committee on Trauma, Eastern Association for the Surgery of Trauma Seniors Committee, Baltimore, Maryland, USA

MOHAMMED IQBAL AHMED, MBBS, FRCA, FAAP
Associate Professor of Anesthesiology, University of Texas Southwestern Medical Center, Staff Cardiac Anesthesiologist, Anesthesiologists for Children, Children's Medical Center and Children's Health System of Texas, Dallas, Texas, USA

CATHERINE M. KUZA, MD
Assistant Professor of Anesthesiology, Department of Anesthesiology and Critical Care, Keck School of Medicine of the University of Southern California, Los Angeles, California, USA

AUTHORS

JENNIFER S. ALBRECHT, PhD
Assistant Professor, Department of Epidemiology and Public Health, University of Maryland School of Medicine, Baltimore, Maryland, USA

REZA ASKARI, MD
Assistant Professor, Department of Surgery, Brigham and Women's Hospital, Harvard Medical School, Boston, Massachusetts, USA

KEVIN P. BLAINE, MD, MPH
Assistant Professor, Department of Anesthesiology, Keck School of Medicine of the University of Southern California, Los Angeles, California, USA; Trauma Anesthesiology Society, Inc, Houston, Texas, USA

RAVI CHAUHAN, FRCA, FCAI, Dip IMC RCSEd
Royal Centre of Defence Medicine, Birmingham, United Kingdom; Division of Trauma Anesthesiology, R Adams Cowley Shock Trauma Center, University of Maryland School of Medicine, Baltimore, Maryland, USA

BIANCA CONTI, MD
Division of Trauma Anesthesiology, R Adams Cowley Shock Trauma Center, University of Maryland School of Medicine, Baltimore, Maryland, USA

MATTHEW D'ANGELO, DNP, CRNA, LTC, USAR, AN
Associate Professor, Assistant Program Director, Nurse Anesthesia Program, Uniformed Services University of the Health Sciences, Daniel K. Inouye Graduate School of Nursing, Bethesda, Maryland, USA

RICHARD P. DUTTON, MD, MBA
Department of Anesthesiology, Texas A&M School of Medicine, US Anesthesia Partners, Dallas, Texas, USA

NABIL M. ELKASSABANY, MD, MSCE
Associate Professor, Department of Anesthesiology and Critical Care, Perelman School of Medicine, University of Pennsylvania, Philadelphia, Pennsylvania, USA

STEPHEN R. ESTIME, MD
Assistant Professor of Anesthesiology, Department of Anesthesiology and Critical Care, The University of Chicago Medicine, Chicago, Illinois, USA

SAMIR FAKHRY, MD
Surgeon, Department of Surgery, Synergy Surgicalists, Inc, Reston Hospital Center, Reston, Virginia, USA

SAMUEL M. GALVAGNO Jr, DO, PhD, FCCM
Associate Professor, Department of Anesthesiology, Program in Trauma, Division Chief, Critical Care Medicine, University of Maryland School of Medicine, Associate Chief Medical Officer, Maryland Critical Care Network, R Adams Cowley Shock Trauma Center, Baltimore, Maryland, USA

KEVIN B. GEROLD, DO, JD
Associate Professor (Retired), Department of Anesthesiology and Critical Care Medicine, Johns Hopkins School of Medicine, Baltimore, Maryland, USA; Tactical EMS Section Chair, National Tactical Officers Association (NTOA), Colorado Springs, Colorado, USA

JESSICA LYNN GROSS, MD, FACS
Assistant Professor, Trauma Surgery, Wake Forest School of Medicine, Wake Forest Baptist Medical Center, Winston-Salem, North Carolina, USA

CATHERINE HEIM, MD, MSc
Department of Anaesthesiology, Center Hospitalier Universitaire Vaudois – CHUV, Lausanne, Switzerland

KENJI INABA, MD
Division of Acute Care Surgery, LAC+USC Medical Center, Los Angeles, California, USA

LEWIS J. KAPLAN, MD
Surgical Services, Professor, Department of Surgery, Division of Trauma, Surgical Critical Care and Emergency Surgery, Hospital of the University of Pennsylvania, Veteran's Administration Medical Center, Corporal Michael J Crescenz VA Medical Center, Perelman School of Medicine, University of Pennsylvania, Philadelphia, Pennsylvania, USA

MICHEL J. KEARNS, MD
Department of Anesthesiology, Naval Medical Center San Diego, Commander, Medical Corps, U.S. Navy, San Diego, California, USA

CATHERINE M. KUZA, MD
Assistant Professor of Anesthesiology, Department of Anesthesiology and Critical Care, Keck School of Medicine of the University of Southern California, Los Angeles, California, USA

MEGHAN B. LANE-FALL, MD, MSHP
Assistant Professor, Department of Anesthesiology and Critical Care, Perelman School of Medicine, Leonard Davis Institute of Health Economics, University of Pennsylvania, Philadelphia, Pennsylvania, USA

JENNIFER K. LEE, MD
Associate Professor, Department of Anesthesiology and Critical Care Medicine, Division of Pediatric Anesthesiology, Johns Hopkins University, Baltimore, Maryland, USA

SARAH A. LEE, MD
Assistant Professor, Department of Anesthesiology, Director of Trauma Anesthesiology Fellowship, University of Washington, Harborview Medical Center, Seattle, Washington, USA

VENKAT REDDY MANGUNTA, MD
Assistant Professor, Department of Anesthesiology, Divisions of Cardiovascular Anesthesia and Critical Care Medicine, Saint Luke's Mid America Heart Institute, University of Missouri-Kansas City School of Medicine, Kansas City, Missouri, USA

EVIE G. MARCOLINI, MD
Assistant Professor, Department of Surgery, Division of Emergency Medicine, University of Vermont College of Medicine, Burlington, Vermont, USA

KAZUHIDE MATSUSHIMA, MD
Division of Acute Care Surgery, LAC+USC Medical Center, Los Angeles, California, USA

JEFFRY T. NAHMIAS, MD, MHPE
Assistant Professor, Department of Surgery, University of California, Irvine, Orange, California, USA

LENA M. NAPOLITANO, MD, FACS, FCCP, MCCM
Professor of Surgery, Division Chief, Acute Care Surgery (Trauma, Burn, Critical Care, Emergency Surgery), Associate Chair, Department of Surgery, Director, Trauma and Surgical Critical Care, University of Michigan Health System, University Hospital, Ann Arbor, Michigan, USA

JAIME ORTIZ, MD
Associate Professor, Department of Anesthesiology, Baylor College of Medicine, Houston, Texas, USA

ALISON R. PERATE, MD
Assistant Professor, Department of Anesthesiology and Critical Care, The Children's Hospital of Philadelphia, Perelman School of Medicine, University of Pennsylvania, Philadelphia, Pennsylvania, USA

EVAN G. PIVALIZZA, MBChB, FFASA
Distinguished Teaching Professor, Department of Anesthesiology, University of Texas McGovern Medical School, Houston, Texas, USA

OLIVER C. RADKE, MD, PhD, DEAA, MHBA
Chair, Department of Anesthesia and Intensive Care Medicine, Klinikum Bremerhaven-Reinkenheide, Bremerhaven, Germany; Associate Adjunct Professor, Department of Anesthesia and Perioperative Care, University of California, San Francisco, San Francisco, California, USA; Professor, Department of Anesthesia, Technical University of Dresden, Dresden, Germany

DAVINDER RAMSINGH, MD
Director of Clinical Research and Perioperative Ultrasound, Associate Professor, Department of Anesthesiology, Loma Linda University School of Medicine, Loma Linda University Medical Center, Loma Linda, California, USA

KINJAL N. SETHURAMAN, MD, MPH
Hyperbaric Medicine-Shock Trauma, Assistant Professor, University of Maryland, Baltimore, Maryland, USA

MANDEEP SINGH, MD
Assistant Professor, Cardiothoracic Anesthesiology and Critical Care, Department of Anesthesiology, Keck Medical Center, University of Southern California, Los Angeles, California, USA

ERIK B. SMITH, MD, JD, MS
Instructor, Department of Anesthesiology and Critical Care Medicine, Division of Pediatric Anesthesiology, Johns Hopkins University, Baltimore, Maryland, USA

CHRISTOPHER T. STEPHENS, MD
Associate Professor, Department of Anesthesiology, University of Texas McGovern Medical School, Houston, Texas, USA

MARC P. STEURER, MD, MHA, DESA
Vice Chief, Department of Anesthesia and Perioperative Care, Zuckerberg San Francisco General Hospital and Trauma Center, Associate Professor, UCSF School of Medicine, San Francisco, California, USA; President-Elect, Trauma Anesthesiology Society, Inc, Houston, Texas, USA

MATTHIAS STOPFKUCHEN-EVANS, MD
Assistant Professor, Department of Anesthesiology, Brigham and Women's Hospital, Harvard Medical School, Boston, Massachusetts, USA

MONICA S. VAVILALA, MD
Professor of Anesthesiology and Pediatrics, Department of Anesthesiology, University of Washington, Director, Harborview Injury Prevention and Research Center, Harborview Medical Center, Seattle, Washington, USA

MATTHEW WELDER, DNP, CRNA, FAWM, DiMM, LTC(ret), USA, AN
Assistant Professor, Uniformed Services University of the Health Sciences, Daniel K. Inouye Graduate School of Nursing, Bethesda, Maryland, USA

DAVID A. YOUNG, MD, MEd, MBA, FAAP
Trauma Committee, Anesthesiology Liaison, Director, Pediatric Anesthesiology Simulation, Medical Director, Pediatric Advanced Life Support Program, Professor, Department of Anesthesiology, Perioperative, and Pain Medicine, Baylor College of Medicine, Texas Children's Hospital, Houston, Texas, USA

Contents

> Monitoring the quality of trauma care is important but particularly challenging. Preventable death assessment aims to identify those cases where the patient's death would have not occurred if the patient had been treated differently. Determination of preventable death in trauma care is often based on calculated probability of survival, commonly by using the Trauma and Injury Severity Score (TRISS). TRISS is not suited for identifying all cases with opportunities for improvement. Combined with other methods such as morbidity and mortality conferences, however, it might be a valid approach if a complete review of all trauma deaths is not feasible at an institution.

> As the principal operating room resuscitationists, anesthesiologists must be familiar with the principles of *Advanced Trauma Life Support®, 10th edition*. This edition recommends a highly structured approach to trauma patients and endorses several advances in trauma resuscitation. There are less stringent guidelines for crystalloid administration, references to video-assisted laryngoscopy, suggested use of viscoelastic methods to guide transfusion decisions, and other changes reflecting recent advances. This article discusses trauma team approach to resuscitation, greater focus on special populations, de-emphasis of spinal immobilization in favor of restriction of spinal motion, and other updates and technical advances.

> Trauma patients who require intubation are at higher risk for aspiration, agitation/combativeness, distorted anatomy, hemodynamic instability, an unstable cervical spine, and complicated injuries. Although rapid-sequence intubation is the most common technique in trauma, slow-sequence intubation may reduce the risk for failed intubation and

cardiovascular collapse. Providers often choose plans with which they are most comfortable. However, developing a flexible team-based approach, through recognition of complicating factors in trauma patients, improves airway management success.

The resuscitation of patients with traumatic hemorrhage remains a challenging clinical scenario. The appropriate and aggressive support of the patient's coagulation is of critical importance. Conventional coagulation assays present several shortcomings in this setting. The integration of viscoelastic monitoring in clinical practice has the potential to result in significant improvements. In order to be successful, the provider must understand basics of the methodology, read outs, and the limitations of the technique.

The incorporation of enhanced recovery after surgery (ERAS) fundamentals into perioperative medicine has improved the patient care experience and hastened recovery time while reducing hospital costs. Research studies have shown that incorporating ERAS principles in the adult or geriatric acute care surgery populations minimizes time to resumption of preoperative activity and reduces hospital length of stay. ERAS principles are widely applicable to these patient cohorts and may be applicable in trauma patients. Increased physician and nursing education to promote widespread utilization of enhanced recovery protocols will further improve quality of health care administered in the twenty-first century.

It is imperative to find the balance between pain control and addressing the opioid epidemic. Opioids, although effective in the acute pain management, have multiple side effects and can lead to dependence, abuse, overdose, or death. Physicians should identify patients who abuse opioids, using their states' prescription drug-monitoring programs and use screening tools to identify patients at increased risk of developing opioid dependence. Multimodal analgesic plans, incorporating regional techniques, and nonopioid medications should be employed to reduce the amount of opioids received by patients.

Caring for the trauma patient requires an in-depth knowledge of the pathophysiology of trauma, the ability to rapidly diagnose and intervene to reverse the derangements caused by shock states, and an aptitude for the use of advanced monitoring techniques and perioperative point-of-care ultrasonography (P-POCUS) to assist in diagnosis and delivery of care. Historically, anesthesiology has lagged behind in wholly embracing this technology. P-POCUS has the potential to allow the trauma anesthesiologist to diagnose numerous injuries, quickly guide the placement of central vascular catheters and invasive monitors, and assess the efficacy of interventions.

Trauma data bank and other research reveal sex disparities in trauma care. Risk-taking behaviors leading to traumatic injury have been associated with sex, menstrual cycle timing, and cortisol levels. Trauma patient treatment stratified by sex reveals differences in access to services at trauma centers as well as specific treatments, such as venous thromboembolism prophylaxis and massive transfusion component ratios. Trauma patient outcomes, such as in-hospital mortality, multiple organ failure, pneumonia, and sepsis are associated with sex disparities in the general trauma patient. Outcome after general trauma and specifically traumatic brain injury show mixed results with respect to sex disparity.

Pediatric traumatic brain injury (TBI) uniquely affects the pediatric population. Abusive head trauma (AHT) is a subset of severe pediatric TBI usually affecting children in the first year of life. AHT is a form of nonaccidental trauma. Sports-related TBI resulting in concussion is a milder form of TBI affecting older children. Current recommended perioperative management of AHT and sports concussions relies on general pediatric TBI guidelines. Research into more specific pediatric TBI screening and management goals is ongoing. This article reviews the epidemiology, mechanisms, clinical signs, and management of AHT and sports-related concussions.

Postintensive care syndrome (PICS) is a heterogeneous syndrome marked by physical, cognitive, and mental health impairments experienced by critical care survivors. It is a syndrome that bears significant human and health care costs. Additional research is needed to identify risk factors and diagnostic, preventative, and treatment strategies for PICS. Trauma intensive care unit patients are particularly vulnerable to posttraumatic stress disorder, which shares some of the adverse long-term consequences of PICS and also requires additional research into effective preventative and management strategies.

combat casualty care, evacuation, fresh whole-blood administration, freeze-dried plasma, and forward surgical care military medicine helped reduce combat mortality to its lowest levels in history. Through the account of a young wounded marine wounded in Iraq, this article examines how innovations on the battlefield saved casualties and explores how these techniques may be applied at home.

ANESTHESIOLOGY CLINICS

RELATED INTEREST

THE CLINICS ARE AVAILABLE ONLINE!
Access your subscription at:
www.theclinics.com

Foreword

Perioperative Care of the Trauma Patient: New Concepts Since Wartime Learning

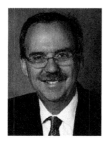

Lee A. Fleisher, MD, FACC, FAHA
Consulting Editor

Trauma care has evolved significantly since its development during wartime, and that includes the role of the anesthesiologist and the influence beyond simple intraoperative resuscitation. In this issue of *Anesthesiology Clinics*, a series of articles has been commissioned that address the acute care, intraoperative management, and long-term implications. As enhanced recovery after surgery has become commonplace for elective surgery, an article on the implications to trauma care has been included. There are also very timely articles on issues of care in the era of the opioid epidemic, long-term implications of care, and hospital planning for an active shooter incident. Finally, the implications of trauma care to home are discussed.

In order to commission an issue on trauma care, I have turned to a former faculty colleague and national expert, Maureen McCunn, MD, MIPP. Maureen is currently Professor of Anesthesiology at the University of Maryland and a member of the Division of Trauma Anesthesiology at the R Adams Cowley Shock Trauma Center. She has leadership roles as a member of the Board of Directors of the Trauma Anesthesiology Society, Chair of the American Society of Anesthesiologists (ASA) Committee on Trauma, and a member of the Eastern Association for the Surgery of Trauma Seniors Committee. She has solicited two outstanding colleagues to assist in editing this issue. Mohammed Iqbal Ahmed, MBBS is Associate Professor of Anesthesiology at the University of Texas Southwestern Medical Center and a Staff Cardiac Anesthesiologist at Children's Medical Center and Children's Health System of Texas. He serves on the ASA Committee on Trauma and Emergency Preparedness and the Society for Pediatric Anesthesia Committee on International Education and Service. Catherine M. Kuza, MD is an Assistant Professor in the Department of Anesthesiology at Keck School of

Anesthesiology Clin 37 (2019) xiii–xiv
https://doi.org/10.1016/j.anclin.2018.11.002
1932-2275/19/© 2018 Published by Elsevier Inc.

Medicine of the University of Southern California. She is a member of the Trauma Anesthesiology Society and has served on the ASA Committee on Trauma and Emergency Preparedness.

Lee A. Fleisher, MD, FACC, FAHA
Perelman School of Medicine
University of Pennsylvania
3400 Spruce Street, Dulles 680
Philadelphia, PA 19104, USA

E-mail address:
Lee.Fleisher@uphs.upenn.edu

Preface

Modern Day Trauma Care for the Anesthesiologist

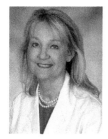
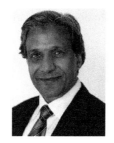
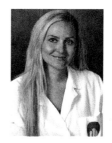

Maureen McCunn, MD, MIPP, FCCM, FASA	Mohammed Iqbal Ahmed, MBBS, FRCA, FAAP	Catherine M. Kuza, MD

Editors

We hope that each of you will find this "cutting-edge" issue of *Anesthesiology Clinics* on trauma-related topics enlightening, thought provoking, and comprehensive. I would like to thank my coeditors, Drs Iqbal Ahmed of the University of Texas and Catherine Kuza of the University of Southern California, for their intense work on bringing this final product to you. In this issue, we have attempted to provide the latest technologies and techniques in modern trauma care and have also included a few "out-of-the-box" topics to make this *Anesthesiology Clinics* issue an inclusive review of trauma care for the anesthesiologist.

We begin with a review of preventable death, performance improvement through morbidity and mortality conferences, and utilization of TRISS methodology. The discussion of the recent ATLS updates will prepare the anesthesiologist for current management priorities of patients following traumatic injury. The review of medications for a "rapid sequence intubation," now referred to in the latest ATLS guidelines as "drug assisted intubation," and the introduction of a "slow sequence intubation" technique for those patients who are hemodynamically unstable, have a possible "difficult airway," or who have complicated medical comorbidities, incorporate general anesthesiology practices into trauma scenarios.

Additional clinically applicable articles are those that deal with the use of viscoelastic testing in hemorrhagic shock, the implementation of enhanced recovery after surgery pathways for emergency and trauma patients, and pain management techniques in the era of the opioid crisis. Point-of-care ultrasound is presented as a critical adjunct for the anesthesiologist to quickly diagnose or rule out injuries and to guide procedures.

We present a unique discussion of the surprising, and conflicting, roles that gender plays on trauma patient outcomes and an article on unique subsets of traumatic brain injury in the pediatric population. We also include an article on post–intensive care

Anesthesiology Clin 37 (2019) xv–xvi
https://doi.org/10.1016/j.anclin.2018.11.001
1932-2275/19/© 2018 Published by Elsevier Inc.

syndrome and describe the associated adverse long-term sequelae seen in trauma survivors, especially those with a prolonged ICU course.

The "cutting-edge" articles of this issue include anesthesiologists' roles in prehospital and in-hospital disaster management as well as in an active shooter event. Newer interventions are discussed, such as resuscitative endovascular balloon occlusion of the aorta, emergency preservation and resuscitation, and resuscitative care interventions employed by US and UK militaries and their associated survival rates. These interventions include advanced technologies for the intervention of severe hemorrhagic shock, the positioning of complementary surgical/anesthesia teams far forward, and the use of whole blood in the field.

Maureen McCunn, MD, MIPP, FCCM, FASA
Department of Anesthesiology
University of Maryland
School of Medicine
Division of Trauma Anesthesiology
R Adams Cowley Shock Trauma Center
22 Greene Street
Baltimore, MD 21201, USA

Mohammed Iqbal Ahmed, MBBS, FRCA, FAAP
University of Texas
Southwestern Medical Center
Children's Medical Center and
Children's Health System of Texas
D2073.03
1935 Medical District Drive
Dallas, TX 75235, USA

Catherine M. Kuza, MD
Department of Anesthesiology and Critical Care
Keck School of Medicine of the University of Southern California
1450 San Pablo Street, Suite 3600
Los Angeles, CA 90033, USA

E-mail addresses:
mmccunn@som.umaryland.edu (M. McCunn)
iqbal.ahmed@childrens.com (M.I. Ahmed)
Catherine.Kuza@med.usc.edu (C.M. Kuza)

Recognizing Preventable Death

Is There a Role of Survival Prediction Algorithms?

Oliver C. Radke, MD, PhD, DEAA, MHBA[a,b,c,*], Catherine Heim, MD, MSc[d]

KEYWORDS

- Preventable death • TRISS • Performance improvement • Trauma • Benchmarking

KEY POINTS

- Interdisciplinary Peer Review is an essential for maintaining and improving quality of care in trauma medicine.
- To lower cost of peer review, one can focus on cases of preventable death, commonly identified by applying Trauma and Injury Severity Score (TRISS) to estimate the probability of survival.
- TRISS is a score that has been in use for more than 30 years; attempts to replace TRISS have failed because TRISS still best predicts survival.
- Limiting cases for peer review to those with supposedly preventable death commonly misses cases with relevant opportunities for process improvement.
- If a review of all trauma deaths is not feasible, combining the preventable death strategy with other methods (ie, CIRS or morbidity and mortality conferences) is necessary.

INTRODUCTION

Everyone involved in trauma care knows that we cannot save every patient. It seems obvious that a patient with a simple ankle fracture should easily survive their injury and that patients presenting with complex and severe polytraumatic injuries and/or

Disclosures: Dr O.C. Radke is a consultant for Draeger medical, Germany and Getinge, Sweden. He received speaker fees from CSL Behring. Dr C. Heim has no disclosures to report.
[a] Department of Anesthesia and Intensive Care Medicine, Klinikum Bremerhaven-Reinkenheide, Postbrookstraße 103, Bremerhaven 27574, Germany; [b] Department of Anesthesia and Perioperative Care, University of California in San Francisco, 1001 Potrero Avenue, San Francisco, CA 94110, USA; [c] Department of Anesthesia, Technical University of Dresden, Fetscherstraße 74, 01307 Dresden, Germany; [d] Department of Anaesthesiology, Center Hospitalier Universitaire Vaudois – CHUV, Rue du Bugnon 21, Vaud, Lausanne CH-1011, Switzerland
* Corresponding author. Department of Anesthesia and Intensive Care Medicine, Klinikum Bremerhaven-Reinkenheide, Postbrookstraße 103, Bremerhaven 27574, Germany.
E-mail address: oradke@pcat.de

1932-2275/19/© 2018 Elsevier Inc. All rights reserved.

requiring cardiopulmonary resuscitation will most likely succumb to their injuries. However, what about those patients presenting in-between these two extremes? Are you confident that you treated all your patients in the best manner possible? And even if *you* did everything perfectly right, what about the rest of your team? What about your trauma surgeons, blood bank, intensive care unit (ICU), and even rehabilitation centers? Did you perform better than other hospitals, had they treated the same patient? And most importantly, is there anything you can (or must) do better in the future?

Medical errors are known to be common, especially in the setting of emergency care for critically ill patients.[1,2] Reports from the early 1990s revealed that a worryingly high percentage of trauma patients do not receive the best standard of care.[3–6] Even amongst designated Level I trauma centers, persisting gaps in quality of trauma care with wide variability in clinical outcomes have been reported.[7,8]

Quality assessment in trauma has been recognized as an issue of utmost importance long before the recent focus on patient safety and health care costs. Dating back to 1961, Van Wagoner was amongst the first to evaluate the quality of care provided to injured patients by applying the concept of preventable death assessment, a method first described in 1933 for maternal care.[9] He found in his report that up to 30% of more than 600 noncombat military deaths resulted either from survivable injuries or in the context of inadequate treatment.[10]

The recognition that trauma deaths might be avoidable in an optimal setting, and if treated in the most adequate manner, has led to the implementation of a systematic approach to trauma care with designation of specialized trauma centers.[11–14] The publication of the landmark report of the Institute of Medicine about medical errors,[15] promoting the adherence to evidence-based strategies, has contributed to the increasing interest in quality assessment and performance monitoring in health care.[16]

Measuring and monitoring the quality of trauma care is particularly challenging because of the complexity of the possible injuries, varying in type and severity in a group of patients that is very heterogeneous in age and preinjury health status. The identification of the optimal method to assess the quality of provided care has been extensively debated over the past few decades. Objective, reproducible, and validated methods are needed in order to measure progress over time within systems and to benchmark the outcomes of one center against others. Today, more than 1500 audit filters and quality indicators are used worldwide.[17] One of most debated quality indicators is the determination of preventable deaths. In this article, the authors discuss the various methods and tools used to assess trauma outcomes and quality of care delivery.

PEER REVIEW OF PREVENTABLE DEATH

Preventable death is generally defined as a death that would have not occurred if an alternative strategy would have been followed or if the patient would have been treated in a different, more optimal setting. Classically, determination of preventable death rate in trauma care is based either on calculated probability of survival or on a peer review of patients' records by a group of experts.[18–23] Preventable death studies have been largely accepted as a standard tool to benchmark trauma care and they have shown to contribute to major improvements in trauma care.[22,24–29] However, evidence for any of the currently published methods assessing quality of trauma care is lacking and there is an ongoing debate about the most reliable, objective, and cost- and resource-effective method. With the enhanced scope of outcome analysis, focusing on not only mortality rates but also functional outcome and cost-effectiveness, interest is growing for in-depth analyses of the entire pathway of care.

Historically, autopsy reports were the basis for early audits in trauma care. However, autopsy reports were criticized for being subjective as initially often performed by a single reviewer. Further criticism was raised because they integrate neither clinical records nor the view of the clinicians involved in cases that were being evaluated.[30] Indeed, later studies have demonstrated that autopsies alone are insufficient for preventable death assessment.[31]

Peer review is an established method for scrutinizing the quality of care in health care settings, both on a systems level (eg, reviewing the standards of care in a single ICU) and on a case-by-case level (eg, reviewing patients' files). The value of the peer review of preventable death assessment in the evaluation of trauma care has been largely accepted, and its evidence of reliability and validity has recently been highlighted.[32] However, its reliability highly depends on the methodology because panel studies have an inherent subjectivity. In a frequently cited comprehensive analysis of reliability of preventable death judgments, many factors have been reported as lowering its reliability such as inclusion criteria and study population characteristics. The case mix of the analyzed population has shown to influence the preventability judgment. Panels are more likely to judge deaths as nonavoidable in patients older than 55 years, in presence of a high Injury Severity Score (ISS), if death occurred within 48 hours or if the cause of death is attributed to injury to the central nervous system. The lack or incompleteness of documentation has shown to influence panel judgment in favor for preventable death.[21] Other factors influencing the validity of peer review are the panel composition and the lack of a clearly stated definition of preventability.[21,23,31,33–37]

If properly designed, expert peer review can generate valuable information on processes and delivered care, and compare the provided care against institutional standards. Sanddal and colleagues provided an example of a thoroughly organized peer review process. In order to obtain the optimal consistency and efficiency of the expert review, they adopted a 3-step plan:

1. Providing the experts with clear guidelines on how to define preventability.
2. All panel members underwent a formal information and training process to be familiarized with the method.
3. Panelists were further provided with a checklist of specific issues to examine.

In addition, in order to ascertain the validity of the reviewers' judgment, the investigators interspersed the patient files with test cases that had previously been reviewed by other panels. Such a careful organization is likely to provide the best possible reliability of the panel review but needs even more extensive resources and a large-scale commitment from the involved clinicians. In a thorough cost analysis, Shackford and colleagues[22] found that on average approximately 1 man-hour is needed for a complete case review by a comprehensive panel. Depending on the volume of cases to be reviewed, this amount of manpower might not be available to every trauma center. In addition, it is unlikely that important information can be obtained by looking at a large mass of average cases; the lessons to be learned are usually found within the cases that are outliers for some reason. Hence the approach to focus on trauma cases of patients who did not survive despite a realistic chance of survival—preventable deaths.

MacKenzie and colleagues[23] reviewed trauma studies evaluating the peer review process. They revealed that the inclusion criteria for the peer review process varied and ranged from including all deaths to only those with a certain degree of severity of injury or after a preselection according to their calculated probability of survival. Panel composition varied from a single reviewer or a purely surgical panel to a large multidisciplinary spectrum, including clinicians and governance stakeholders. Decision-making strategies were done by consensus or majority vote, but in up to one-third of studies this important element was not reported. Probably one of the most important flaws, rendering these preventable death studies greatly incomparable, is the lack of a standardized definition of "preventability." Most studies did not provide their reviewers with clear guidelines about how to judge "preventability." Frames of reference for preventability judgment went from "according to the clinicians expertise,"[38] "if this patient would have been admitted to a fully staffed and equipped American style trauma center"[39] to "if injury occurred in front of the hospital."[40] Amongst the 19 studies with explicit guidelines 9 different versions could be identified with only a maximum of 4 using the same variants. Therefore, criteria for preventability ranged from completely implicit to extensively defined.

Despite its successful application, peer review is criticized for its dependence on the reviewers' subjective judgment. Furthermore, the workload needed to review clinical records of all trauma deaths (and the large volume of trauma patients) makes this method difficult to implement for many centers. In addition, when the American Professional Standards Review Organizations (PSRO) Act[41] was created in order to establish a national review process of medical care, it provoked considerable concern and skepticism with the clinicians who saw the PSRO as "agents for cost containment."[42,43] Consequently, several studies attempted to identify alternative tools to assess trauma outcomes that are more objective, reliable, reproducible, and less time- and resource-consuming. Algorithms based on scores seem to be most promising to fulfill these requirements.[19]

TRAUMA OUTCOME ASSESSMENT TOOLS
Trauma and Injury Severity Score

In 1987, Boyd and colleagues[19] developed an approach to evaluate the quality of trauma care based on a statistical calculation: the TRISS methodology. TRISS calculates the probability of survival of a particular patient based on the physiologic compromise to the severity of injury, and it takes into account the mechanism of injury as well as the patient's age. Nonsurviving trauma patients with a TRISS value (ie, probability of survival) of greater than 50% are classified as "unexpected deaths."

This statistical approach promised to overcome the subjectivity of peer review. It gained wide acceptance as an objective and less time-consuming measure of outcome and performance. The TRISS method became a standard for trauma care evaluation and is used for ranking hospital performance and monitoring preventable mortality rates.[19,44,45] However, its superiority to peer review has never been demonstrated, and other, more comprehensive scores have been developed.

The TRISS method estimates a trauma patient's survival probability by relating the degree of physiologic compromise as determined by the Revised Trauma Score (RTS)[46] to the extent of anatomic injury as expressed by the ISS.[47] Further integrated variables are mechanism of injury and the patient's age. In the original study, TRISS values were related to survival probability by logistic regression data based on a small cohort of a single center. Published in 1990, the American College of Surgeons' Major Trauma Outcome Study (MTOS),[20] which evaluated more than 80,000 patients, provided a comprehensive overview of outcomes in injured patients. The purposes of MTOS were to develop national norms for trauma care so that trauma centers could measure their outcome as compared with the MTOS norm, based on the management of injuries of similar extent. MTOS was the first multicenter database used to derive TRISS norms from that moment on, TRISS-based calculation of probability of survival has been widely used as an outcome prediction model for trauma patients. Further more, it has been suggested as an "audit filter" to identify patients with unexpected outcomes.[48] The concept of statistically "expected" versus "unexpected death," determined conventionally by a TRISS-Probability of survival (TRISS-Ps) threshold of 50%, has been proposed for patient selection worthy for review in mortality au-dits.[18–20] This threshold, however, is empiric and the accuracy between the patients' identified unexpected death-rates and preventability as assessed by experts is un-clear.[21,49,50] The extent of missing elements of preventability and opportunities for improvement by not reviewing the "expected deaths" is unknown. Some centers even use the TRISS-methodology to completely replace the preventable death approach.[34]

Trauma and Injury Severity Score Limitations

Unfortunately, TRISS has a range of well-documented limitations, questioning its value for the evaluation of trauma outcomes. TRISS is calculated from the ISS and components of the RTS, which include the type of injury and physiologic parameters (ie, Glasgow Coma Scale, systolic blood pressure, respiratory rate, etc.). The physiologic parameters (especially respiratory rate) are often missing. It has been shown that more data are missing in patients who are more likely to die, and most databases have more missing TRISS components for patients who die than for survivors.[51] This seems to be an increasing phenomenon. The MTOS-study had 11.3% of missing data needed for TRISS-calculation; the recent national sample project of the American National Trauma Data Bank has reportedly up to 22.4% missing items.[45] With the advances in prehospital care, most severely injured patients arrive intubated to the trauma center and the patient's own respiratory rate can therefore not be assessed.

The ISS is a measure of the severity of physical injury and is derived from the Abbre-viated Injury Scale (AIS), which scores the severity of injury from a scale of 1 to 6 for 6 specified body regions. The sum of the squares of the 3 highest AIS scores is used to calculate ISS and it ranges from 1 to 75.[52] ISS is subject to a certain degree of observer bias because it depends on capture of injuries by registry personnel and may vary depending on the skills and experience of the coder. As ISS takes only the most severe injuries per body region into account,[53,54] the severity of patients with multiple injuries in the same body region may be underestimated and therefore overestimate TRISS-based probability of survival.

TRISS is commonly criticized for being derived from a study based on the North American trauma population, which might affect its validity in other settings as for example in the European area with a substantially lower proportion of penetrating trauma. De Jongh and colleagues[55] showed that the MTOS-based model performed adequately in a homogenous setting of patients but that the discriminative power of TRISS in patients with "minor injuries with hip fractures" was close to "coincidence."

Trauma Mortality Prediction Model

The Trauma Mortality Prediction Model (TMPM-ICD9) is a survival prediction based on patients' ICD-9 codes,[56] which factors in patients' preexisting medical conditions (ie, congestive heart failure, cerebrovascular accident, etc.), which may significantly in-crease mortality.[57] The failure to incorporate comorbid conditions is a limitation of TRISS. However, TMPM-ICD9 failed to outperform TRISS.[58]

Kim and colleagues[59] increased the receiver operating characteristic curve (ROC) of TRISS significantly by incorporating the serum albumin level at admission, a very elegant approach because serum albumin is a known surrogate for multiple chronic conditions, and hypoalbuminemia is generally associated with poorer outcomes. It also has the advantage of being absolutely objective, whereas ICD-9 codes will be biased depending on the coder's experience and the risk of upcoding when trying to optimize reimbursement by payers. On the other hand, ICD-9 codes are readily available, whereas injury scores and laboratory values might be missing from patient records, hence precluding appropriate calculation of survival with TRISS.

TRISS estimates the probability of survival based on linear statistical models. One might question whether these models are actually suited to analyze complex biological systems such as a human being. Nevertheless, using advanced artificial intelligence technologies such as neural networks to calculate the probability of survival did not surpass the performance of the established method[60] but was a close second. Perhaps this method can demonstrate advantages further on, especially when fed with more data points, and a well-trained neural network could also be more robust when dealing with missing data.[61] Either way, to assume that patients with "expected death" as determined by a TRISS threshold of less than 50% do not present any elements of preventability or opportunities for improvement in either the clinical care or the system setting means neglecting the uncertainty of outcome prediction. Patients with a TRISS less than 50% still have ∼50% chance of survival and TRISS scores in middle ranges (25%–75%) are known to have the greatest inconsistency in reliability. The TRISS-based definition of "unexpected death" has therefore been questioned.[62–64]

Despite these limitations, TRISS continues to be the gold standard tool for benchmarking purposes in trauma outcomes[65] and has even been used to predict future performance of trauma centers based on historic data.[65] A TRISS threshold of 50% has been identified as significant "yield" for peer review process, as advocated notably by the American Surgical College Committee on Trauma.[5,66] Seven studies in this review were conducted with the aim to assess the validity of a preselection of patients for peer review done by TRISS. Therefore, only patients with "unexpected death" were subjected to peer review. Agreement rates were then evaluated between peer review and TRISS-based judgment. Takanayagi and colleagues[67] stated that TRISS overestimates the preventable death rate and Phair and colleagues[68] found a poor agreement between TRISS-identified preventable death and those assigned by peer review. Karmy-Jones and colleagues[49] estimated that TRISS selection, despite limitations, "provides a basis for reliable, consistent peer review process." This is similar to the conclusions of Cayten and colleagues,[69] who estimated that TRISS alone is insufficient for preventable death assignment, but it may be useful as an audit filter to "strengthen the conclusion of preventable death studies." However, these studies did not examine the rate of preventable deaths amongst the "expected death," which might have influenced their judgment, because it has been shown that elements of preventability can be found at all TRISS levels.[64,70] Gruen and colleagues[71] limited their peer review process by deaths with TRISS greater than 50%, but they included patients with identified issues in a morbidity and mortality (M&M) conference, which reviewed every of the 2594 trauma deaths in the study. This procedure identified an additional 53 patients in "need" of review. Such procedures might eventually be as valuable as reviewing all trauma deaths, depending on the composition of M&M conferences and discussed documents. In their study however, M&M meetings are described as "surgical" — multidisciplinary meetings would potentially enhance the reliability of identification of elements of preventability.[21]

In 2016, a study group from London evaluated the TRISS method in a very large real-life sample of trauma patients.[72] They included data from more than 14,000 traumas

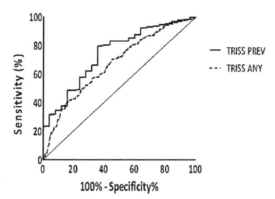

Fig. 1. Receiver operating curves for TRISS. ROC curve of the predictive capacity of TRISS for preventable deaths ("TRISS PREV"; AUC 0.74, CI: 0.64–0.83) and any preventability ("TRISS ANY"; AUC 0.66, CI: 0.62–0.71). (*From* Heim C, Cole E, West A, et al. Survival prediction algorithms miss significant opportunities for improvement if used for case selection in trauma quality improvement programs. Injury 2016;47(9):1964; with permission.)

that occurred over an 8-year period (2006–2013). The study population had an overall mortality of 5.6%, and after excluding cases with missing data, 626 trauma death cases were reviewed manually. About 30% (190 cases) had some elements of preventability, whereas 25 deaths were deemed to have been preventable (4%).

Following the manual review and classification, the investigators tried to find the best TRISS score threshold to reliably identify cases of preventable death. For instance, with a threshold of 75%, only 30% of the trauma deaths would have been classified as unexpected. Although this would greatly reduce the workload of the review panel, the reviewers would have missed more than half of the preventability issues that had been found by the review of all the trauma deaths. The ROC of the predictive capacity of TRISS for preventable deaths had an area under the curve of only 0.74 and even lower (0.66) for any preventable issues (**Fig. 1**).

SUMMARY

There is no perfect tool or algorithm to predict trauma survival and outcomes. However, TRISS is a fairly reliable tool to predict survival after trauma, and is deemed to be the gold standard. Reliable as it is for a reasonably large sample of patients, TRISS is not suited for identifying all cases of preventable death, with opportunities for performance improvement. Combining the TRISS score with other methods, such as identifying specific patient factors in M and M conferences, may strengthen the predictive ability of this tool. Using TRISS to identify cases relevant for peer review may be a valid approach if a complete review of all trauma deaths is not feasible at an institution, but the reviewers will most likely miss at least half of the opportunities for performance improvement. We do advocate therefore for a thorough review of *all* trauma deaths in a standardized, multidisciplinary review process.

REFERENCES

1. Hoyt DB, Hollingsworth-Fridlund P, Fortlage D, et al. An evaluation of provider-related and disease-related morbidity in a level I university trauma service: directions for quality improvement. J Trauma 1992;33(4):586–601.

2. Davis JW, Hoyt DB, McArdle MS, et al. The significance of critical care errors in causing preventable death in trauma patients in a trauma system. J Trauma 1991; 31(6):813–8 [discussion: 818–9].

3. Copes WS, Staz CF, Konvolinka CW, et al. American College of Surgeons audit filters: associations with patient outcome and resource utilization. J Trauma 1995;38(3):432–8.

4. Nayduch D, Moylan J, Snyder BL, et al. American College of Surgeons trauma quality indicators: an analysis of outcome in a statewide trauma registry. J Trauma 1994;37(4):565–73 [discussion: 573–5].

5. Rhodes M, Sacco W, Smith S, et al. Cost effectiveness of trauma quality assurance audit filters. J Trauma 1990;30(6):724–7.

6. O'Keefe GE, Jurkovich GJ, Maier RV. Defining excess resource utilization and identifying associated factors for trauma victims. J Trauma 1999;46(3):473–8.

7. Glance LG, Osler TM, Dick AW, et al. The Survival Measurement and Reporting Trial for Trauma (SMARTT): background and study design. J Trauma 2010; 68(6):1491–7.

8. Glance LG, Dick AW, Meredith JW, et al. Variation in hospital complication rates and failure-to-rescue for trauma patients. Ann Surg 2011;253(4):811–6.

9. New York Academy Medicine. Maternal mortality in New York city; a study of all puerperal deaths, 1930-1932. New York; London: Commonwealth fund, H. Milford, Oxford University Press; 1933.

10. Van Wagoner FH. A three year study of deaths following trauma. J Trauma 1961;1: 401–8.

11. Boyd DR. A symposium on The Illinois Trauma Program: a systems approach to the care of the critically injured. Introduction: a controlled systems approach to trauma patient care. J Trauma 1973;13(4):275–6.

12. Gill W, Champion HR, Long WB, et al. A clinical experience of major multiple trauma in Maryland. Md State Med J 1976;25(1):55–8.

13. Waters JM Jr, Wells CH. The effects of a modern emergency medical care system in reducing automobile crash deaths. J Trauma 1973;13(7):645–7.

14. West JG, Trunkey DD, Lim RC. Systems of trauma care. A study of two counties. Arch Surg 1979;114(4):455–60.

15. Institute of Medicine. To err is human: building a safer health system. Washington, DC: The National Academies Press; 2000.

16. Werner RM, Bradlow ET. Relationship between Medicare's hospital compare performance measures and mortality rates. JAMA 2006;296(22):2694–702.

17. Stelfox HT, Bobranska-Artiuch B, Nathens A, et al. Quality indicators for evaluating trauma care: a scoping review. Arch Surg 2010;145(3):286–95.

18. Champion HR, Sacco WJ, Hunt TK. Trauma severity scoring to predict mortality. World J Surg 1983;7(1):4–11.

19. Boyd CR, Tolson MA, Copes WS. Evaluating trauma care: the TRISS method. Trauma score and the injury severity score. J Trauma 1987;27(4):370–8.

20. Champion HR, Copes WS, Sacco WJ, et al. The Major Trauma Outcome Study: establishing national norms for trauma care. J Trauma 1990;30(11):1356–65.

21. MacKenzie EJ, Steinwachs DM, Bone LR, et al. Inter-rater reliability of preventable death judgments. The Preventable Death Study Group. J Trauma 1992; 33(2):292–302 [discussion: 302–3].

22. Shackford SR, Hollingsworth-Fridlund P, McArdle M, et al. Assuring quality in a trauma system–the Medical Audit Committee: composition, cost, and results. J Trauma 1987;27(8):866–75.

23. MacKenzie EJ. Review of evidence regarding trauma system effectiveness resulting from panel studies. J Trauma 1999;47(3 Suppl):S34–41.
24. West JG, Cales RH, Gazzaniga AB. Impact of regionalization. The Orange County experience. Arch Surg 1983;118(6):740–4.
25. Spain DM, Fox RI, Marcus A. Evaluation of hospital care in one trauma care system. Am J Public Health 1984;74(10):1122–5.
26. Cales RH, Trunkey DD. Preventable trauma deaths. A review of trauma care systems development. JAMA 1985;254(8):1059–63.
27. Kreis DJ Jr, Plasencia G, Augenstein D, et al. Preventable trauma deaths: Dade County, Florida. J Trauma 1986;26(7):649–54.
28. Shackford SR, Hollingworth-Fridlund P, Cooper GF, et al. The effect of regionalization upon the quality of trauma care as assessed by concurrent audit before and after institution of a trauma system: a preliminary report. J Trauma 1986; 26(9):812–20.
29. Cales RH. Trauma mortality in Orange County: the effect of implementation of a regional trauma system. Ann Emerg Med 1984;13(1):1–10.
30. Mosberg WH. Trauma centers and truth in advertising. Neurosurgery 1980;7(2): 191–4.
31. West JG. Validation of autopsy method for evaluating trauma care. Arch Surg 1982;117(8):1033–5.
32. Stelfox HT, Straus SE, Nathens A, et al. Evidence for quality indicators to evaluate adult trauma care: a systematic review. Crit Care Med 2011;39(4):846–59.
33. McDermott FT, Cordner SM, Tremayne AB. Reproducibility of preventable death judgments and problem identification in 60 consecutive road trauma fatalities in Victoria, Australia. Consultative Committee on Road Traffic Fatalities in Victoria. J Trauma 1997;43(5):831–9.
34. Sampalis JS, Boukas S, Nikolis A, et al. Preventable death classification: interrater reliability and comparison with ISS-based survival probability estimates. Accid Anal Prev 1995;27(2):199–206.
35. Esposito TJ, Sanddal ND, Hansen JD, et al. Analysis of preventable trauma deaths and inappropriate trauma care in a rural state. J Trauma 1995;39(5): 955–62.
36. Maio RF, Burney RE, Gregor MA, et al. A study of preventable trauma mortality in rural Michigan. J Trauma 1996;41(1):83–90.
37. Wilson DS, McElligott J, Fielding LP. Identification of preventable trauma deaths: confounded inquiries? J Trauma 1992;32(1):45–51.
38. Hill DA, Lennox AF, Neil MJ, et al. Evaluation of TRISS as a means of selecting trauma deaths for clinical peer review. Aust N Z J Surg 1992;62(3):204–8.
39. Anderson ID, Woodford M, de Dombal FT, et al. Retrospective study of 1000 deaths from injury in England and Wales. Br Med J (Clin Res Ed) 1988; 296(6632):1305–8.
40. Stocchetti N, Pagliarini G, Gennari M, et al. Trauma care in Italy: evidence of in-hospital preventable deaths. J Trauma 1994;36(3):401–5.
41. Smits HL. The PSRO in perspective. N Engl J Med 1981;305(5):253–9.
42. Dans PE, Weiner JP, Otter SE. Peer review organizations. Promises and potential pitfalls. N Engl J Med 1985;313(10):1101–7.
43. Rutstein DD, Berenberg W, Chalmers TC, et al. Measuring the quality of medical care. A clinical method. N Engl J Med 1976;294(11):582–8.
44. Llullaku SS, Hyseni NS, Bytyçi CI, et al. Evaluation of trauma care using TRISS method: the role of adjusted misclassification rate and adjusted w-statistic. World J Emerg Surg 2009;4:2.

45. Schluter PJ. Trauma and Injury Severity Score (TRISS): is it time for variable re-categorisations and re-characterisations? Injury 2011;42(1):83–9.
46. Champion HR, Sacco WJ, Copes WS, et al. A revision of the trauma score. J Trauma 1989;29(5):623–9.
47. Baker SP, O'Neill B, Haddon W Jr, et al. The injury severity score: a method for describing patients with multiple injuries and evaluating emergency care. J Trauma 1974;14(3):187–96.
48. Copes WS, Champion HR, Sacco WJ, et al. Progress in characterizing anatomic injury. J Trauma 1990;30(10):1200–7.
49. Karmy-Jones R, Copes WS, Champion HR, et al. Results of a multi-institutional outcome assessment: results of a structured peer review of TRISS-designated unexpected outcomes. J Trauma 1992;32(2):196–203.
50. Gillott AR, Copes WS, Langan E, et al. TRISS unexpected survivors–a statistical phenomenon or a clinical reality? J Trauma 1992;33(5):743–8.
51. Gabbe BJ, Cameron PA, Wolfe R. TRISS: does it get better than this? Acad Emerg Med 2004;11(2):181–6.
52. Rating the severity of tissue damage. I. The abbreviated scale. JAMA 1971; 215(2):277–80.
53. Younge PA, Coats TJ, Gurney D, et al. Interpretation of the Ws statistic: application to an integrated trauma system. J Trauma 1997;43(3):511–5.
54. Champion HR, Copes WS, Sacco WJ, et al. Improved predictions from a severity characterization of trauma (ASCOT) over Trauma and Injury Severity Score (TRISS): results of an independent evaluation. J Trauma 1996;40(1):42–8 [discussion: 48–9].
55. de Jongh MA, Verhofstad MH, Leenen LP. Accuracy of different survival prediction models in a trauma population. Br J Surg 2010;97(12):1805–13.
56. Glance LG, Osler TM, Mukamel DB, et al. TMPM-ICD9: a trauma mortality prediction model based on ICD-9-CM codes. Ann Surg 2009;249(6):1032–9.
57. Benjamin ER, Khor D, Cho J, et al. The age of undertriage: current trauma triage criteria underestimate the role of age and comorbidities in early mortality. J Emerg Med 2018;55(2):278–87.
58. Akay S, Ozturk AM, Akay H. Comparison of modified Kampala trauma score with trauma mortality prediction model and trauma-injury severity score: a National Trauma Data Bank Study. Am J Emerg Med 2017;35(8):1056–9.
59. Kim SC, Kim DH, Kim TY, et al. The Revised Trauma Score plus serum albumin level improves the prediction of mortality in trauma patients. Am J Emerg Med 2017;35(12):1882–6.
60. Becalick DC, Coats TJ. Comparison of artificial intelligence techniques with UK-TRISS for estimating probability of survival after trauma. UK Trauma and Injury Severity Score. J Trauma 2001;51(1):123–33.
61. Rubin DB, Little RJA. Statistical analysis with missing data. 2nd edition. New York: Wiley; 2002.
62. Zoltie N, de Dombal FT. The hit and miss of ISS and TRISS. Yorkshire Trauma Audit Group. BMJ 1993;307(6909):906–9.
63. Norris R, Woods R, Harbrecht B, et al. TRISS unexpected survivors: an outdated standard? J Trauma 2002;52(2):229–34.
64. Kelly AM, Nicholl J, Turner J. Determining the most effective level of TRISS-derived probability of survival for use as an audit filter. Emerg Med (Fremantle) 2002;14(2):146–52.
65. Glance LG, Mukamel DB, Osler TM, et al. Ranking trauma center quality: can past performance predict future performance? Ann Surg 2014;259(4):682–6.

66. Resources for optimal care of the injured patient: an update. Task Force of the Committee on Trauma, American College of Surgeons. Bull Am Coll Surg 1990; 75(9):20–9.

67. Takayanagi K, Koseki K, Aruga T. Preventable trauma deaths: evaluation by peer review and a guide for quality improvement. Emergency Medical Study Group for Quality. Clin Perform Qual Health Care 1998;6(4):163–7.

68. Phair IC, Barton DJ, Barnes MR, et al. Deaths following trauma: an audit of performance. Ann R Coll Surg Engl 1991;73(1):53–7.

69. Cayten CG, Stahl WM, Agarwal N, et al. Analyses of preventable deaths by mechanism of injury among 13,500 trauma admissions. Ann Surg 1991;214(4): 510–20 [discussion: 520–1].

70. Shanti CM, Tyburski JG, Rishell KB, et al. Correlation of revised trauma score and injury severity score (TRISS) predicted probability of survival with peer-reviewed determination of trauma deaths. Am Surg 2003;69(3):257–60 [discussion: 260].

71. Gruen RL, Jurkovich GJ, McIntyre LK, et al. Patterns of errors contributing to trauma mortality: lessons learned from 2,594 deaths. Ann Surg 2006;244(3): 371–80.

72. Heim C, Cole E, West A, et al. Survival prediction algorithms miss significant opportunities for improvement if used for case selection in trauma quality improvement programs. Injury 2016;47(9):1960–5.

Advanced Trauma Life Support® Update 2019
Management and Applications for Adults and Special Populations

Samuel M. Galvagno Jr, DO, PhD[a],*, Jeffry T. Nahmias, MD, MHPE[b],
David A. Young, MD, MEd, MBA[c]

KEYWORDS

- Advanced Trauma Life Support® • ATLS® • Trauma resuscitation
- Damage control resuscitation • Damage control surgery • Trauma anesthesiology
- Trauma • Injuries

KEY POINTS

- *Advanced Trauma Life Support®, 10th edition (ATLS®-10)* endorses several advances in trauma resuscitation that anesthesiologists must be familiar with.
- Trends (rather than absolute values of vital signs) and base excess figure prominently in an updated classification scheme for hemorrhagic shock.
- The updated version of the Glasgow Coma Scale has been simplified; pressure, rather than pain, is used to illicit abnormal responses.
- *ATLS®-10* recommends use of a short-acting beta blocker (ie, esmolol) to decrease the heart rate to less than 80 beats per minute and targets a mean arterial pressure of 60 to 70 mm Hg when managing traumatic aortic dissection.
- In special populations, there are numerous anesthetic considerations that must be considered.

Disclosure Statement: All authors (S.M. Galvagno, J.T. Nahmias, D.A. Young) are certified instructors for the American College of Surgeons (ACS) Advanced Trauma Life Support® Course. As such, a small stipend is paid to each for teaching, depending on the segments of the course taught, in accordance with the practices of the Committee on Trauma for the ACS. The authors have no other relationships with any commercial entities that have a direct financial interest in the subject matter and materials discussed in this article.

[a] Department of Anesthesiology, Program in Trauma, Critical Care Medicine, University of Maryland School of Medicine, Maryland Critical Care Network, R Adams Cowley Shock Trauma Center, 22 South Greene Street, T3N08, Baltimore, MD 21201, USA; [b] Department of Surgery, University of California, Irvine, 101 the City Drive South, Building 1, Orange, CA 92868, USA; [c] Trauma Committee, Anesthesiology Liaison, Pediatric Anesthesiology Simulation, Pediatric Advanced Life Support Program, Department of Anesthesiology, Perioperative, and Pain Medicine, Baylor College of Medicine, Texas Children's Hospital, 6621 Fannin Street Suite A-3300, Houston, TX 77030, USA
* Corresponding author.
E-mail address: sgalvagno@som.umaryland.edu

Anesthesiology Clin 37 (2019) 13–32
https://doi.org/10.1016/j.anclin.2018.09.009
1932-2275/19/© 2018 Elsevier Inc. All rights reserved.

INTRODUCTION

The Advanced Trauma Life Support® (ATLS®) course was developed in 1978 by the American College of Surgeons, and its accompanying textbook, *Advanced Trauma Life Support, 10th edition (ATLS®-10)*, was updated in 2018.[1] ATLS® is the most broadly disseminated and recognized training program for the initial assessment, stabilization, and management of the injured patient worldwide. As the principal resuscitationists in the operating room, anesthesiologists must be familiar with the principles of ATLS®. This article discusses the application of ATLS® principles for adult trauma patients, as well as some special patient populations, including children. Although a summary of recent changes to *ATLS®-10* are discussed here, a comprehensive review of the ATLS® course is impracticable because an entire textbook is devoted to the topic.

OVERVIEW OF *ADVANCED TRAUMA LIFE SUPPORT, 10TH EDITION*

ATLS®-10 promotes numerous revisions to previous dogmatic practices in trauma, including less stringent guidelines for crystalloid administration (ie, the previous mandatory 2 L of crystalloids before considering transfusion is no longer supported), references to video-assisted laryngoscopy, the suggested use of viscoelastic methods (ie, TEG™ and ROTEM™) to guide transfusion decisions, and many other changes that reflect recent advances in trauma resuscitation. *ATLS®-10* emphasizes the concept of a trauma team approach to resuscitation, a greater focus on special populations (eg, the elderly, obese persons), a de-emphasis on spinal immobilization in favor of restriction of spinal motion, and several other updates and technical advances, which are discussed in the sections that follow.

INITIAL ASSESSMENT

A structured and systematically performed primary survey is the foundation for the initial assessment of the trauma patient.[1] The primary survey uses a mnemonic for the sequential management priorities of airway, breathing, circulation, and disability (ABCD). The ABCD survey should be repeated frequently and whenever a patient's status changes. The secondary survey occurs after the primary survey is complete and the patient's vital functions are improving. The secondary survey involves a head-to-toe examination and documenting all abnormal findings, while protecting the patient from hypothermia. The elements of the primary and secondary survey are described in **Boxes 1** and **2**.

AIRWAY MANAGEMENT

The term rapid sequence intubation has been removed from *ATLS®-10* and replaced with the term drug-assisted intubation. From an anesthesiologist's perspective, use of this new term is rather unsuitable because the process of rapid sequence induction and intubation is the preferred term used by most trauma anesthesiologists and endorsed by major trauma societies.[2–5] Ambiguous terminology notwithstanding, the principles of early definitive airway management are well-understood by anesthesiologists and are discussed in greater depth elsewhere.[2,6] *ATLS®-10* defines a definitive airway as the presence of a cuffed tube in the trachea, achieved either by endotracheal or nasotracheal intubation, cricothyrotomy, or tracheostomy.[1] Airway management in the trauma patient, unlike current guidelines for advanced cardiac life support, remains the crucial first step in the management of a trauma patient. (See Stephen R. Estime and Catherine M. Kuza's article, "Trauma Airway Management: Induction Agents, Rapid Versus Slower Sequence Intubations, and Special Considerations," discussion of some airway management issues, in this issue.)

Box 1
Primary ATLS® survey

Primary survey

Step 1. Don personal protective equipment, assign team roles

Step 2. Assess (*A*) *airway* patency, including examination of the neck and thorax for signs of a pneumothorax or hemothorax.
- During the airway assessment, the Glasgow Coma Scale (GCS) score may be assessed to determine if the patient can protect the airway; a GCS ≤ 8 usually indicates the need for endotracheal intubation.
- Cervical motion restriction should be maintained if injury is suspected.
- NEXUS criteria: if there is no midline tenderness, no neurological deficits, no distracting injury, no altered mental status or intoxication, C-spine radiographs are not required.

The airway should be managed definitively if not considered secure; ATLS® defines a definitive airway as a cuffed tube in the trachea.

Step 3. Assess (*B*) *breathing* adequacy. Determine if the patient is spontaneously breathing. Assess skin color, chest rise and fall, and rate and depth of respirations. Assess soft tissue and bony chest wall integrity. Auscultate breath sounds. Apply supplemental oxygen or transition to mechanical ventilation if airway is secure.
- Potential interventions: needle chest decompression, finger thoracostomy, thoracostomy tube placement

Obtain a chest radiograph and/or lung ultrasound examination (eFAST).

Step 4. Assess (*C*) *circulation.* Assess pulse rate and character both peripherally and centrally. Obtain blood pressure. Focus on identifying sources of hemorrhage, including external as well as cavitary sources.
- Potential interventions: placement of large-bore intravenous catheters, wound packing, application of combat application tourniquet, application of traction splints, placement of an intraosseous device, application of pelvic binder, ultrasound-guided pericardiocentesis, administration of fluid, transfusion of blood products

Note: If intra-abdominal hemorrhage is strongly suspected, it is reasonable to perform an eFAST examination at this stage.

Step 5. Assess (*D*) *disability.* Perform a brief neurological examination, including calculating the GCS score, pupil examination, and examination for lateralizing signs.
- Potential interventions: head/spine radiograph (including computed tomography except in cases in which urgent transfer would be delayed) interpretation, implementation of cervical spine imaging decision tools (NEXUS and Canadian rules), restrict spine movement (remove backboard as soon as possible), remove helmet

Protect against hypothermia (eg, warm blankets, warm fluids, remove wet clothes)

Step 6. Proceed with secondary survey

Abbreviations: ATLS, advanced trauma life support; eFAST, extended focused assessment with sonography in trauma.
    Adapted from 10th Edition of the Advanced Trauma Life Support® (ATLS®) Student Course Manual, 2018. American College of Surgeons, Chicago, IL.

SHOCK

In *ATLS®-10*, a new classification scheme is presented for the 4 classes of hemorrhagic shock; this is among the most significant updates since the inception of the ATLS® program (**Table 1**).[1]

The updated classification recognizes the shortcomings of previous iterations and includes a category for pulse pressure and base deficit because both have been shown to correlate highly with the degree of hypovolemia due to

---

Box 2
Secondary ATLS® survey

Secondary survey

Step 1. Obtain AMPLE history from patient, family, or prehospital personnel.
  A- Allergies
  M- Medications
  P- Past history, illnesses, pregnancies
  L- Last meal
  E- Environment and exposure

Step 2. Obtain history of injury-producing event and identify mechanisms of injury.

Step 3. Assess the head and maxillofacial area.

Step 4. Assess the cervical spine and neck.
• Inspect for signs of blunt and penetrating injury, tracheal deviation, and use of accessory respiratory muscles
• Palpate for tenderness, deformity, swelling, subcutaneous emphysema, tracheal deviation, symmetry of pulses
• Auscultate the carotid arteries for bruits
• Restrict cervical spinal motion if injury suspected

Step 5. Assess the chest.
• Inspect all aspects for signs of blunt and penetrating injury
• Auscultate lung fields and assess quality of respiratory excursions and/or use of accessory muscles
• Percuss for evidence of hyperresonance or dullness

Step 6. Assess the abdomen.
  Inspect, auscultate, percuss, and palpate the abdomen looking for signs of blunt or penetrating injuries and signs of internal bleeding

Step 7. Assess the perineum/rectum/vagina.
• Only perform a rectal examination in selected patients (ie, when looking for blood, bony fragments, assessing anal sphincter tone in cases of spinal injury, or assessing bowel wall integrity)
• Perform a vaginal assessment in selected patients
• Look for contusions, hematomas, and lacerations in the perineum
• Assess for urethral bleeding

Step 8. Perform a musculoskeletal assessment.
• Inspect and palpate upper and lower extremities for signs of blunt and penetrating injury
• Assess the pelvis for evidence of fracture and associated hemorrhage
• Palpate all peripheral pulses
• Inspect and palpate the thoracic and lumbar spines (while restricting spinal motion in patients with possible spinal injury)

Step 9. Perform a neurological assessment.
• Reevaluate the pupils
• Determine the Glasgow Coma Scale score
• Evaluate upper and lower extremities for motor and sensory function
• Observe for lateralizing signs (ie, paresis, plegia, hyperreflexia)

Abbreviation: ATLS, advanced trauma life support.
  Adapted from 10th Edition of the Advanced Trauma Life Support® (ATLS®) Student Course Manual, 2018. American College of Surgeons, Chicago, IL.

---

hemorrhage.[7,8] Importantly, trends, not absolute values, are emphasized to assist clinicians with estimating blood loss and transfusion requirements. In patients with class I or II hemorrhage, fluid resuscitation with up to 1 L of warm saline is recommended. Early resuscitation with blood and blood products (not additional

Table 1				
Updated Advanced Trauma Life Support classification for hemorrhagic shock				
Parameter	Class I	Class II (Mild)	Class III (Moderate)	Class IV (Severe)
Approximate blood loss	<15%	15%–30%	31%–40%	>40%
Heart rate	↔	↔/↑	↑	↑/↑↑
Blood pressure	↔	↔	↔/↓	↓
Pulse pressure	↔	↓	↓	↓
Respiratory rate	↔	↔	↔/↑	↑
Urine output	↔	↔	↓	↓↓
GCS score	GCS score ↔	GCS score ↔	GCS score ↓	GCS score ↓↓
Base deficit	0 to −2 mEq/L	−2 to −6 mEq/L	−6 to −10 mEq/L	−10 mEq/L or more
Need for blood products	Monitor	Possible	Yes	Massive transfusion

From American College of Surgeons. Advanced trauma life support. 10th edition. Chicago: American College of Surgeons, Committee on Trauma; 2018; with permission.

crystalloid or colloid) is advised in patients with evidence of class II or greater hemorrhage.[9] Early administration of blood products at a low ratio (ie, 1 U packed red blood cells to 1 U fresh frozen plasma to 1 U platelets) can prevent development of coagulopathy and thrombocytopenia.[1,10] Additional updates in *ATLS®-10* include discussions about the requirement for large-bore (18 gauge or larger) intravenous access, use of intraosseous access devices,[11,12] early application of tourniquets, management of patients receiving novel anticoagulants,[13,14] and use of hemostatic adjuncts (eg, tranexamic acid and prothrombin concentrates). Viscoelastic assays, such as TEG™ or ROTEM™, are also cited as potentially helpful diagnostic aids.

TRAUMATIC BRAIN INJURY

In 2016, the Brain Trauma Foundation published updated guidelines for the management of severe traumatic brain injury (TBI).[15] These guidelines, among others,[16] are referenced in *ATLS®-10*, and a summary of anesthesia-related considerations for TBI patients is detailed in **Table 2**.

The Glasgow Coma Scale (GCS) is a valuable tool for assessing TBI, and an updated version is endorsed in the *ATLS®-10* (**Table 3**).[1,17]

In the updated GCS, eye opening to pressure, rather than pain, is described and 3 sites for physical stimulation are recommended (ie, fingertip pressure, trapezius pinch, supraorbital notch pressure). For the verbal component, the terms inappropriate words and incomprehensible sounds have been simplified to words and sounds. For the motor component assessment, the term withdrawal has been removed and replaced with normal and abnormal flexion. Abnormal flexion responses to physical stimulation include slow stereotyped movements, movement of the arm across the chest (rather than movement of the arm away from the body), rotation of the forearm, clenching of the thumb, or leg extension. When aspects of the GCS assessment cannot be completed (eg, when a patient is intubated), the untestable component is designated as not testable (NT).

Table 2
Summary of anesthetic considerations based on the 2016 Brain Injury Foundation guidelines for the management of severe traumatic brain injury

Phase	Parameter or Modality	Recommendation or Comment	Anesthetic Consideration
Treatment	Hyperosmolar therapy	• Hyperosmolar therapy with mannitol or hypertonic saline may lower intracranial pressure (ICP) but there is insufficient evidence to support the use of 1 rather than the other.	Hyperosmolar agents are often required preoperatively and intraoperatively. When using mannitol, the anesthetist must be aware of fluid shifts; hypovolemia in a patient with concurrent hemorrhagic shock can be exacerbated.
	CSF	• An external ventricular device (EVD) zeroed at the midbrain with continuous drainage of CSF may be considered to lower ICP; this may be more effective than intermittent use. • The use of an EVD to lower ICP in patients with an initial GCS <6 during the first 12 h of injury may be considered.	Continuous monitoring requires constant intraoperative vigilance; excessive drainage can lead to brain herniation.
	Ventilation therapies	• Hyperventilation is recommended as a temporizing measure for the reduction of elevated ICP. • Hyperventilation should be avoided during the first 24 h after injury when cerebral blood flow (CBF) is often critically reduced. • Prolonged hyperventilation with a $Paco_2$ of 25 mm Hg of less is not recommended.	The target $Paco_2$ is 35–45 mm Hg; $Paco_2$ is a powerful determinant of CBF. Low $Paco_2$ levels result in low CBF and cerebral ischemia, whereas high $PaCO_2$ levels can result in cerebral hyperemia and high ICP.
	Anesthetics, analgesics, sedatives	• The use of barbiturates to induce burst suppression as measured by EEG because prophylaxis against an elevated ICP is not recommended. • High-dose barbiturate administration is recommended to control elevated ICP refractory to maximum standard medical and surgical treatment. • Propofol is recommended to help control ICP but caution is required because high-dose propofol is associated with significant morbidity.	Patients with ICP elevation refractory to standard medical treatment may present to the operating room on a barbiturate infusion. High-dose propofol should be avoided.

Steroids	• The use of steroids is not recommended. High-dose methylprednisolone is associated with increased mortality.	Steroids are contraindicated and should not be administered in the operating room.
Infection prophylaxis	• General critical care protocols and practices should be followed to prevent ventilator-associated pneumonia; periprocedural antibiotics for intubation are no longer recommended.	Antibiotics before intubation are not required (a change from the previous ATLS®, 3rd edition, guidelines).
Seizure prophylaxis	• Early (within 7 d of injury) administration of phenytoin is recommended to decrease the incidence of posttraumatic seizures. • There is insufficient evidence to recommend levetiracetam (Keppra) over phenytoin regarding efficacy in preventing posttraumatic seizures.	Seizure prophylaxis with phenytoin is often initiated in the operating room. Active seizures should be treated per the standard of care (ie, midazolam or lorazepam).
Prophylactic hypothermia	• Not recommended to improve outcomes in patients with diffuse injury.	Temperature monitoring for TBI patients is mandatory; normothermia should be maintained.
Monitoring ICP monitoring	• Management of severe TBI patients using information from ICP monitoring is recommended to reduce postinjury mortality.	Although not supported by evidence meeting current standards, ICP should be measured in TBI patients with a GCS of 3–8 and an abnormal CT scan (ie, revealing hematomas, contusions, swelling, herniation, or compressed basal cisterns). ICP monitoring may also be indicated in severe TBI patients with a normal CT scan who are older than 40 y, have hypotension (SBP <90 mm Hg), or exhibit unilateral or bilateral motor posturing.
Cerebral perfusion pressure (CPP) monitoring	• CPP monitoring is recommended to decrease mortality.	CPP is proportional to the gradient between MAP and mean ICP; MAP can be modulated directly by the anesthetist (ie, vasopressors, fluids) and requires close monitoring (ie, arterial catheter) and treatment in the operating room.
Advanced cerebral monitoring	• Jugular bulb monitoring of arteriovenous oxygen content difference may be considered. • Brain tissue oxygen monitoring is no longer recommended owing to insufficient evidence.	Anesthetists should be aware of the presence of jugular bulb monitors and how to correctly interpret the information provided by these devices.

(continued on next page)

Table 2
(continued)

Phase	Parameter or Modality	Recommendation or Comment	Anesthetic Consideration
Thresholds	Blood pressure	• Maintaining SBP ≥100 mm Hg for patients 50–69 y or at ≥110 mm Hg for patients 15–49 y or >70 y may be considered to decrease mortality and improve outcomes.	Monitoring blood pressure (ie, arterial catheter) and avoiding hypotension in patients with severe TBI is a major perioperative goal.
	ICP	• Treatment of ICP >22 mm Hg is recommended because values above this level are associated with increased mortality.	In practice, a combination of ICP values, clinical examination, and brain CT findings are required to make management decisions.
	CPP	• The recommended CPP value is between 60 and 70 mm Hg.	The exact threshold for CPP is unclear, and depends on the patient's autoregulatory status.
	Advanced monitoring	• A jugular venous saturation <50% may be a threshold to avoid to reduce mortality and improve outcomes.	Anesthetists should be aware of the presence of jugular bulb monitors, and how to correctly interpret the information provided by these devices.

Abbreviations: EEG, electroencephalograph; MAP, mean arterial pressure; PaO2, partial pressure of oxygen; PaCO2, partial pressure of carbon dioxide; SBP, systolic blood pressure.

Adapted from Carney N, Totten AM, O'Reilly C, et al. Guidelines for the management of severe traumatic brain injury, fourth edition. Neurosurgery 2017;80(1):6–15; with permission.

Table 3	
The Glasgow structured approach to assessment of the Glasgow Coma Scale	
Eyes	Spontaneous: 4
	To sound: 3
	To pressure: 2
	None: 1
	Not testable (NT)
Verbal	Oriented: 5
	Confused: 4
	Words: 3
	Sounds: 2
	None: 1
	NT
Motor	Obeys commands: 6
	Localizes: 5
	Normal flexion: 4
	Abnormal flexion: 3
	Extension: 2
	None: 1
	NT

Adapted from Institute of Neurological Sciences NHS Greater Glasgow and Clyde. Glasgow Coma Scale: do it this way. Available at: http://www.glasgowcomascale.org/downloads/GCS-Assessment-Aid-English.pdf?v=3. Accessed September 13, 2018; with permission.

SPINAL CORD INJURY

The use of spinal immobilization is de-emphasized in *ATLS®-10* in favor of an emphasis on restriction of spinal motion.[1] Clinicians are encouraged to remove backboards as soon as practicable because pressure ulcers are common and may develop rapidly in patients with spinal cord injuries.[18] The Canadian C-spine Rule[19] and the National Emergency X-Radiography Utilization Study (NEXUS)[20] criteria are endorsed because both have excellent predictive value for excluding patients identified at low risk for having a cervical spine injury.

Use of these rules may help decrease unnecessary radiological testing and, in the case of anesthesia and airway management, may facilitate easier intubation because cervical spinal motion restriction (ie, cervical collars) can be discontinued safely in many patients. These rules are summarized in **Table 4**.

THORACIC TRAUMA

Blunt chest trauma occurs in greater than 10% of all trauma patients worldwide with mortality rates ranging from 4% to 20%.[21] Immediate life-threatening chest injuries include tension pneumothorax, massive hemothorax, and thoracic aortic injury. Tension pneumothorax is particularly lethal and has historically been implicated in up to 5% of all major trauma patients.[22–24] Physical examination findings to help distinguish between tension pneumothorax and massive hemothorax include percussion, tracheal deviation, and the evaluation of the neck veins. Tension pneumothorax demonstrates hyperresonance, deviation of the trachea away from the injury (a late sign), and distended neck veins. Conversely, a massive hemothorax is associated with dullness to percussion, midline tracheal position, and collapsed neck veins due to hemorrhagic shock.

Table 4
Summary of Canadian and National Emergency X-Radiography Utilization Study cervical spine rules for ruling out injury to the cervical spine

Canadian	NEXUS
High-risk factors that mandate radiography: • Age >65 y • Dangerous mechanism[a] • Paresthesias in extremities	Criteria: • No posterior midline cervical spine tenderness • No evidence of intoxication • Normal level of alertness • No focal neurologic deficits • No painful distracting injuries
Radiography necessary before removal of cervical collar	*Radiography not necessary if previous conditions met*
Low-risk factors that allow safe range of motion assessment: • Simple rear-end motor vehicle crash • Sitting position in the emergency department • Ambulatory (anytime) • Delayed onset of neck pain • No midline cervical tenderness	
Range of motion: • Can rotate neck actively 45° to the right and left	
Radiography not necessary if previous conditions met and cervical collar may be removed	

[a] Fall from greater than 3 feet (1 m or 5 stairs), axial load to the head, motor vehicle crash with high speed, ejection, or rollover, motorized recreational vehicle or bike collision.

Data from Stiell IG, Wells GA, Vandemheen KL, et al. The Canadian C-spine rule for radiography in alert and stable trauma patients. JAMA 2001;286(15):1841–8; and Hoffman JR, Mower WR, Wolfson AB, et al. Validity of a set of clinical criteria to rule out injury to the cervical spine in patients with blunt trauma. National emergency X-radiography utilization study group. N Engl J Med 2000;343(2):94–9.

For the treatment of any hemothorax, *ATLS®-10* previously recommended placement of a large-bore tube thoracostomy. Recent studies have demonstrated that the diameter (size) of the tube does not affect the ability to evacuate a fresh traumatic hemothorax.[25] Therefore, *ATLS®-10* now recommends placement of a smaller 28F to 32F chest tube for any acute hemothorax that is visible on chest radiograph. The treatment of a tension pneumothorax can be accomplished either by tube thoracostomy or, in prehospital situations, needle decompression, which was previously recommended at the midclavicular line of the second intercostal space. A recent systematic review and meta-analysis comparing the midclavicular site to an anterior axillary site found the anterior axillary location to be more favorable in terms of depth (3.42 cm vs 4.28 cm), leading to the ATLS® program adopting this as the preferred location for needle decompression of a pneumothorax.[25–28]

Another immediate life-threatening injury is a blunt thoracic aortic injury. If no contraindication exists, *ATLS®-10* now recommends use of a short-acting beta blocker (ie, esmolol) to decrease the heart rate to less than 80 beats per minute and targets a mean arterial pressure of 60 to 70 mm Hg, with the goal of reducing the risk for rupture or worsening of an existing dissection.[1]

ABDOMINAL TRAUMA

Abdominal and pelvic trauma previously comprised blunt and penetrating trauma. In *ATLS®-10*, an additional distinction is now made regarding blast mechanisms. Physical examination for pelvic injuries previously included evaluation for urethral injury by inspecting for blood at the urethral meatus and performing a rectal examination to evaluate for a high-riding prostate. However, *ATLS®-10* has now removed rectal examination for this purpose due to the poor sensitivity (2%) demonstrated for this maneuver.[29] Additionally, the treatment of severe pelvic fractures with associated hemorrhage has evolved with the advent of preperitoneal pelvic packing,[30] which was recently demonstrated in a single-center study to reduce time to intervention and achieve a lower mortality (21% vs 32%) compared with a large modern series using angioembolization as the initial treatment of hemorrhage control.[31] **Fig. 1** illustrates an approach to pelvic fractures associated with shock.

Anesthesiologists should be familiar with this management approach for resuscitation planning and management of these patients in either the operating room or interventional radiology suite.

MUSCULOSKELETAL TRAUMA

Although most musculoskeletal trauma is not immediately life-threatening, a femur fracture may be associated with enough hemorrhage to cause hemorrhagic shock; hence, the principles of early stabilization and operative repair are emphasized. In

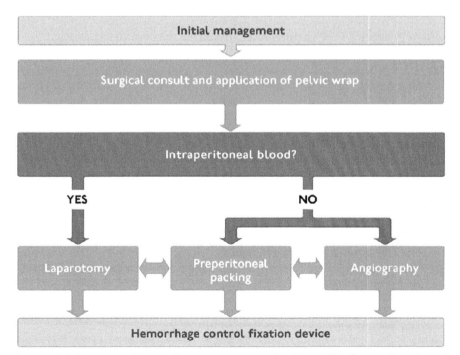

Fig. 1. Pelvic fracture and hemorrhage management algorithm. DPL, diagnostic peritoneal lavage; FAST, focused assessment with sonography in trauma. (*Data from* American College of Surgeons. Advanced trauma life support. 10th edition. Chicago: American College of Surgeons, Committee on Trauma; 2018.)

ATLS®-10, increased vigilance is recommended in the setting of bilateral femur fractures because there is up to an 80% risk of significant associated injuries that may be life-threatening.[32,33]

The administration of prophylactic antibiotics has been proven in multiple previous studies and is incorporated in current guidelines.[34] Furthermore, *ATLS®-10* endorses use of antibiotic prophylaxis for open fractures, recommending weight-based dosing to ensure appropriate levels of the antibiotic are achieved.

THERMAL INJURIES

Burn resuscitation continues to evolve from the days of Charles Baxter[35] and the creation of the Parkland formula in the 1960s. The Parkland formula recommends administration of crystalloid at a rate of 4 mL/kg of percent of total body surface area (TBSA) burned with half of the total fluid volume administered during the first 8 hours from time of injury. This formula initially addressed the serious issue of inadequate resuscitation.[36] However, overaggressive resuscitation has led to an increased incidence of volume overload and development of abdominal compartment syndrome.[37] Therefore, in *ATLS®-10*, use of the modified Brooke Formula is advocated. This formula estimates volume needs as 2 mL/kg of percent of TBSA for burns of at least 20%. Half of the crystalloid is given over the first 8 hours and the rest over the second 16 hours. In conjunction with the American Burn Association Practice Guidelines, *ATLS®-10* now recommends that, regardless of solution type or estimated need, fluids should be titrated to a goal of 0.5 to 1.0 mL/kg/h of urine output and boluses should be avoided unless necessary (eg, hypotension).[36,38]

TRAUMA IN SPECIAL POPULATIONS AND ADVANCED TRAUMA LIFE SUPPORT APPLICATIONS
Pediatric Trauma

Traumatic injuries to children are the most common cause of death and disability in the United States for children older than 1 year of age, accounting for approximately 10,000 deaths yearly.[39] Approximately 10 million children are brought to emergency departments yearly for treatment of injuries.[40] Many injuries occurring in children are preventable; this strengthens the importance of comprehensive injury prevention programs. The most common cause of death in children is motor vehicle incidents[41]; this may be as a passenger or a pedestrian. Other, less common, causes of death in decreasing order include drowning, fires, homicides, and falls. Nonaccidental trauma accounts for almost all homicides in infants.[42] In pediatric patients, falls account for most injuries that are not life-threatening.

Pediatric patients have the following injury characteristics[43]:

- Most injuries result from blunt trauma.
- Blunt trauma can be frequently managed without surgical intervention or with the use of angioembolization.
- Head injury is the most common cause of death and associated hypotension is uncommon (excluding infants); infants have additional protective areas (open fontanelles) to allow expanding intracranial masses.
- Rib fractures are less likely to occur due to incomplete calcification; therefore, significant thoracic force can be transmitted, resulting in a pulmonary contusion or tension pneumothorax.
- Psychological ramifications in the patient and family should be strongly considered.

- Significant blood loss can occur ($\leq$30% of total blood volume) before hypotension may manifest.
- Pseudosubluxation of the cervical spine can be difficult to distinguish from a true injury.
- Ligamentous injuries to the spine occur more commonly in children and can only be definitively diagnosed by MRI.

In general, the management for the pediatric trauma patient will follow a similar approach and use the same ATLS® principles as used for other patients. However, pediatric patients have unique anatomic and physiologic characteristics that result in specific anesthetic implications (**Table 5**).

Applicable content within *ATLS®-10* includes[1]:

- Minimize patient exposure to ionizing radiation by using amounts as low as reasonably achievable.
- Nonaccidental trauma occurs in the pediatric population and should be considered if suggestive history and physical findings are present. (See Smith and colleagues' article, "Pediatric Traumatic Brain Injury and Associated Topics: An Overview of Abusive Head Trauma, Nonaccidental Trauma, and Sports Concussions," in this issue.)
- Use the dislodgement, obstruction, pneumothorax, equipment failure (DOPE) mnemonic to troubleshoot common causes of deterioration in intubated patients.
- There is no change in location for needle decompression of the chest in children (in contrast to adults); this will still occur at the intersection of the second intercostal space and the midclavicular line.
- Intraosseous line placement should be considered if 2 unsuccessful attempts at percutaneous vascular access have occurred.
- Damage control resuscitation is performed by administration of a 20 mL/kg bolus of an isotonic crystalloid solution, followed by balanced ratios of packed red blood cells, plasma, and platelets. This strategy has been implemented within the adult

Table 5
Anatomic and physiologic characteristics of pediatric trauma patients with their respective anesthetic implications

Anatomic or Physiologic Characteristics	Anesthetic Implications
Airway: Relatively large head, increased intraoral tissues, larynx funnel shaped, vocal cords more cephalad and anteriorly located	More likely to develop airway obstruction, require jaw-thrust maneuver, and difficult to obtain a secured airway
Breathing: Increased oxygen consumption (weight-based) and decreased functional residual capacity (weight-based)	Increased rate for development of hypoxemia
Circulation: Cardiac output is rate-dependent, large amount of volume loss possible before blood pressure changes	Bradycardia can contribute to poor perfusion; 30%–40% of blood loss can occur before hypotension develops
Neurologic: Patients may be preverbal due to age and/or developmental limitations	May make standard GCS inappropriate; consider use of pediatric modified GCS
Environmental: Patients likely to have decreased muscle mass and fat stores	Patients at increased risk for development of hypothermia

Data from American College of Surgeons. Advanced trauma life support. 10th edition. Chicago: American College of Surgeons, Committee on Trauma; 2018.

population; however, this strategy has not has been universally applied to the pediatric population owing to lack of data demonstrating a survival advantage.

Geriatric Trauma

According to the Centers for Disease Control and Prevention, the average life expectancy in 2015 in the United States has increased to 78.8 years.[44] The United States Census Bureau has reported that the nation's median age continues to increase; residents aged 65 years and older grew from 35.0 million in 2000, to 49.2 million in 2016.[45] These findings suggest a growing number of geriatric patients and the potential for increased traumatic injuries within this population. It is important to emphasize that the geriatric population has significantly increased mortality for similar injury severities when compared with a younger cohort. This has been postulated to occur owing to multiple factors, including improper triage, senescence of organ systems, and preexisting medical conditions.[46] It is important to consider preexisting medical conditions in the geriatric population as potential causes of traumatic injuries (eg, primary myocardial infarction resulting in a motor vehicle incident).

Within the geriatric population, injury is the fifth leading cause of death. The mechanisms of injury in decreasing order are falls, motor vehicle incidents, burns, and penetrating injuries.[47] Falls are the most common mechanism of injury overall and most likely to result in a fatal outcome within the geriatric population. Motor vehicle incidents and burns within the geriatric population are attributed to multiple causes, including decreased reaction times, limited mobility, and possible cognitive impairment.[48] Blunt trauma is the predominant mechanism of trauma; however, penetrating injuries are the fourth most common cause of death in patients older than 65 years, with many of these related to intentional actions.[49]

In general, the management for the geriatric trauma patient follows a similar approach and uses the same ATLS® principles as used for other patients. Geriatric patients have unique anatomic and physiologic characteristics that result in specific anesthetic implications (**Table 6**).

Applicable content within the *ATLS®-10* includes[1]:

- Geriatric patients have longer hospital stays and less return to independent lifestyles than younger cohorts.
- Five conditions that seem to influence outcome in geriatric trauma patients are cirrhosis, congenital coagulopathy, chronic obstructive pulmonary disease, ischemic heart disease, and diabetes mellitus. Patients with 1 or more of these preexisting conditions are twice as likely to die as those without.
- Mortality from pelvic fractures are 4 times higher in older than younger patients.
- Geriatric patients are more likely to develop rib fractures due to reduced bone density and may subsequently acquire pneumonia.
- Geriatric patients have the highest risk for TBI-associated morbidity and mortality, mostly due to preexisting conditions and associated medications (eg, antiplatelet, anticoagulants).
- Maltreatment occurs in the geriatric population and should be considered if suggestive history and physical findings are present.

Trauma in Pregnancy

Traumatic injuries have been estimated to occur in approximately 6% to 8% of all pregnant patients.[50] Motor vehicle incidents are the most likely mechanism of injury for pregnant trauma patients, followed by falls, assaults, gunshot wounds, and burns. Blunt injuries are much more likely to occur than penetrating ones.[51]

Table 6
Anatomic and physiologic characteristics of geriatric trauma patients with their respective anesthetic implications

Anatomic or Physiologic Characteristics	Anesthetic Implications
Airway: Neck extension may be limited and dentures could be present	May be more likely to develop airway obstruction if edentulous; may be challenging to obtain a secured airway
Breathing: Preexisting conditions (eg, chronic obstructive pulmonary disease) could be present, reduced gas exchange, cough reflex, mucociliary function	Increased risk for hypoxemia, increased work of breathing, and perioperative pneumonia
Circulation: Preexisting conditions and medications (ie, atrial fibrillation, beta blockers) could be present; decreased sensitivity to catecholamines, fixed cardiac output, atherosclerosis	Refractory response to vasoactive medications, increased risk for cardiac ischemia and/or arrhythmias; cardiovascular and pulmonary responses to hypoxemia and/or hypercarbia diminish with age
Neurologic: Patients may have preexisting conditions (ie, Alzheimer disease) and/or developmental limitations	May make use of GCS challenging; postoperative delirium and cognitive dysfunction are higher; general anesthetic requirements are decreased
Environmental: Patients likely to have decreased muscle mass and fat stores; osteoporosis	Patients at increased risk for development of fractures, hypothermia and decubitus ulcers
Other: Renal function decreased	Medication dose adjustment may be required; increased risk of renal injury

Data from American College of Surgeons. Advanced trauma life support. 10th edition. Chicago: American College of Surgeons, Committee on Trauma; 2018.

When caring for the gravid patient with traumatic injuries, it should be appreciated that pregnancy causes significant anatomic and physiologic changes that result in specific anesthetic implications, as well as several notable changes to the expected laboratory values (**Table 7**).

In general, the management of the pregnant trauma patient will follow a similar approach and use the same ATLS® principles as used for other patients. Health care providers appreciate that there are 2 distinct patients; however, they should generally focus efforts on resuscitation of the mother, which will be conveyed to the fetus. The main cause of fetal death is not direct fetal trauma but maternal shock.[52] Obstetric consultation should occur early for the evaluation and management of the pregnant trauma patient.[53]

Applicable content within the *ATLS®-10* includes[1]:

- Vena cava compression from the uterus can significantly decrease cardiac output. This is mitigated by placing the patient in a slight left lateral decubitus position (or elevating the right side of a spine board).
- The uterus remains intrapelvic until 12 weeks of gestation, by 20 weeks it is at the umbilicus, and by 34 weeks it is at the coastal margin.
- As the uterus enlarges, bowel is pushed cephalad, making it somewhat protected from blunt abdominal trauma.
- Fetal heart tones should be continuously monitored after 20 to 24 weeks gestation.

Table 7
Anatomic and physiologic characteristics of pregnant trauma patients with their respective anesthetic implications

Anatomic or Physiologic Characteristics	Anesthetic Implications
Airway: Increased mucosal engorgement of nasal and oral cavities	Increased risk for difficult mask ventilation and tracheal intubation
Breathing: Increased minute ventilation mostly from increased tidal volume; hypocapnia present; increased oxygen consumption, decreased functional residual capacity	Increased risk to develop respiratory distress and hypoxemia
Circulation: Heart rate and cardiac output increased; decreased vascular resistance and blood pressure; plasma volume increased	Increased tolerance from hypovolemia due to delivery; resting tachycardia present; vena cava compression can cause hypotension
Neurologic: Preexisting conditions may be present (ie, epilepsy, eclampsia)	Eclampsia can be challenging to differentiate from TBI; decreased anesthetic requirements (inhalational agents)
Environmental: Uterus can significantly decrease venous return	Position patient in a left lateral decubitus position (or elevate the right side of a spine board).
Other: Several laboratory values altered due to pregnancy	Decreased hematocrit and platelets, increased white blood cells and clotting factors
Delayed gastric emptying	Increased risk for gastric regurgitation and pulmonary aspiration of gastric contents

Data from American College of Surgeons. Advanced trauma life support. 10th edition. Chicago: American College of Surgeons, Committee on Trauma; 2018.

- Amniotic fluid entering intravascularly can result in an amniotic fluid embolism and disseminated intravascular coagulation.
- Fluid in the vagina with a pH greater than 4.5 suggests ruptured chorioamniotic membranes.
- Eclampsia can be diagnostically challenging to differentiate from TBI.
- Perimortem caesarian sections may be successful if performed early for cases of maternal traumatic cardiac arrest.
- Maltreatment occurs in the pregnant population and should be considered if suggestive history and physical findings are present.
- Immunoglobulin therapy (Rho[D] immune globulin) should be given to all Rh-negative mothers unless the injury sites are remote from the abdomen.

TRANSFER TO DEFINITIVE CARE

Despite previous attention to the issue of delays in transfer for definitive care, studies have continued to demonstrate that a significant portion of trauma transfers undergo computed tomography (CT) imaging before transport, which has been shown to lead to delays of an average of 90 minutes.[54] Additionally, multiple studies have demonstrated the high rate of repeat CT scans performed at receiving facilities, which is associated with increased health care costs and radiation exposure for patients.[55,56] For these reasons, *ATLS®-10* places greater emphasis on the need to transfer to definitive care before performing imaging that will not immediately change management. In addition, *ATLS®-10* recommends use of the standardized communication tool of situation, background, assessment, and recommendation (SBAR). Situation information includes the patient's name, age, intravenous access, fluids received, indication for transfer, and the name of the referring physician. Background information includes history of the trauma event, blood products received, imaging performed, past medical or surgical history, medications, and allergies. Assessment information includes vital signs, pertinent examination findings, and patient response to treatments or interventions. Finally, a recommendation for transport mode (ie, helicopter vs ground) and interventions that will be required on arrival should be conveyed.

SUMMARY

ATLS®-10 recommends a highly structured approach to trauma patients. It endorses several advances in trauma resuscitation and provides numerous updated recommendations. The authors strongly advise completion of the ATLS® course for any anesthesiologist appointed to take care of trauma patients.

REFERENCES

1. 10th Edition of the Advanced Trauma Life Support® (ATLS®) Student Course Manual. Chicago (IL): American College of Surgeons; 2018.
2. Dunham CM, Barraco RD, Clark DE, et al. Guidelines for emergency tracheal intubation immediately after traumatic injury. J Trauma 2003;55:162–79.
3. Bassett MD, Smith CE. General anesthesia for trauma. In: Varon AJ, Smith CE, editors. Essentials of trauma anesthesia. New York: Cambridge University Press; 2012. p. 76–94.
4. El-Orbany M, Connolly LA. Rapid sequence induction and intubation: current controversy. Anesth Analg 2010;110:1318–25.
5. Stollings JL, Diedrich DA, Oyen LJ, et al. Rapid-sequence intubation: a review of the process and considerations when choosing medications. Ann Pharmacother 2014;48:62–76.
6. Jain U, McCunn M, Smith CE, et al. Management of the traumatized airway. Anesthesiology 2016;124:199–206.
7. Mutschler M, Nienaber U, Brockamp T, et al. Renaissance of base deficit for the initial assessment of trauma patients: a base deficit-based classification for hypovolemic shock developed on data from 16,305 patients derived from the TraumaRegister DGU(R). Crit Care 2013;17:R42.
8. Mutschler M, Nienaber U, Brockamp T, et al. A critical reappraisal of the ATLS classification of hypovolaemic shock: does it really reflect clinical reality? Resuscitation 2013;84:309–13.
9. Shrestha B, Holcomb JB, Camp EA, et al. Damage-control resuscitation increases successful nonoperative management rates and survival after severe blunt liver injury. J Trauma Acute Care Surg 2015;78:336–41.
10. Holcomb JB, Fox EE, Wade CE, et al. The prospective observational multicenter major trauma transfusion (PROMMTT) study. J Trauma Acute Care Surg 2013;75: S1–2.
11. Lee PM, Lee C, Rattner P, et al. Intraosseous versus central venous catheter utilization and performance during inpatient medical emergencies. Crit Care Med 2015;43:1233–8.
12. Lewis P, Wright C. Saving the critically injured trauma patient: a retrospective analysis of 1000 uses of intraosseous access. Emerg Med J 2015;32:463–7.

13. Baumann Kreuziger LM, Keenan JC, Morton CT, et al. Management of the bleeding patient receiving new oral anticoagulants: a role for prothrombin complex concentrates. Biomed Res Int 2014;2014:583794.
14. Hoffman M, Monroe DM. Reversing targeted oral anticoagulants. Hematology Am Soc Hematol Educ Program 2014;2014:518–23.
15. Carney N, Totten AM, O'Reilly C, et al. Guidelines for the management of severe traumatic brain injury, fourth edition. Neurosurgery 2017;80:6–15.
16. Badjatia N, Carney N, Crocco TJ, et al. Guidelines for prehospital management of traumatic brain injury 2nd edition. Prehosp Emerg Care 2008;12(Suppl 1):S1–52.
17. Teasdale G, ALlen D, Brennan P, et al. The Glasgow Coma Scale: an update after 40 years. Nurs Times 2014;110:12–6.
18. Ham W, Schoonhoven L, Schuurmans MJ, et al. Pressure ulcers from spinal immobilization in trauma patients: a systematic review. J Trauma Acute Care Surg 2014;76:1131–41.
19. Stiell IG, Wells GA, Vandemheen KL, et al. The Canadian C-spine rule for radiography in alert and stable trauma patients. JAMA 2001;286:1841–8.
20. Hoffman JR, Mower WR, Wolfson AB, et al. Validity of a set of clinical criteria to rule out injury to the cervical spine in patients with blunt trauma. National emergency X-radiography utilization study group. N Engl J Med 2000;343:94–9.
21. Battle CE, Hutchings H, Evans PA. Risk factors that predict mortality in patients with blunt chest wall trauma: a systematic review and meta-analysis. Injury 2012;43:8–17.
22. McPherson JJ, Feigin DS, Bellamy RF. Prevalence of tension pneumothorax in fatally wounded combat casualties. J Trauma 2006;60:573–8.
23. Leigh-Smith S, Harris T. Tension pneumothorax–time for a re-think? Emerg Med J 2005;22:8–16.
24. Ivey KM, White CE, Wallum TE, et al. Thoracic injuries in US combat casualties: a 10-year review of operation enduring freedom and Iraqi freedom. J Trauma Acute Care Surg 2012;73:S514–9.
25. Inaba K, Lustenberger T, Recinos G, et al. Does size matter? A prospective analysis of 28-32 versus 36-40 French chest tube size in trauma. J Trauma Acute Care Surg 2012;72:422–7.
26. Laan DV, Vu TD, Thiels CA, et al. Chest wall thickness and decompression failure: a systematic review and meta-analysis comparing anatomic locations in needle thoracostomy. Injury 2016;47:797–804.
27. Leatherman ML, Held JM, Fluke LM, et al. Relative device stability of anterior versus axillary needle decompression for tension pneumothorax during casualty movement: preliminary analysis of a human cadaver model. J Trauma Acute Care Surg 2017;83:S136–41.
28. Powers WF, Clancy TV, Adams A, et al. Proper catheter selection for needle thoracostomy: a height and weight-based criteria. Injury 2014;45:107–11.
29. Ball CG, Jafri SM, Kirkpatrick AW, et al. Traumatic urethral injuries: does the digital rectal examination really help us? Injury 2009;40:984–6.
30. Cothren CC, Osborn PM, Moore EE, et al. Preperitonal pelvic packing for hemodynamically unstable pelvic fractures: a paradigm shift. J Trauma 2007;62:834–9 [discussion: 9–42].
31. Burlew CC, Moore EE, Stahel PF, et al. Preperitoneal pelvic packing reduces mortality in patients with life-threatening hemorrhage due to unstable pelvic fractures. J Trauma Acute Care Surg 2017;82:233–42.

32. Willett K, Al-Khateeb H, Kotnis R, et al. Risk of mortality: the relationship with associated injuries and fracture treatment methods in patients with unilateral or bilateral femoral shaft fractures. J Trauma 2010;69:405–10.

33. Kobbe P, Micansky F, Lichte P, et al. Increased morbidity and mortality after bilateral femoral shaft fractures: myth or reality in the era of damage control? Injury 2013;44:221–5.

34. Hoff WS, Bonadies JA, Cachecho R, et al. East (EAST?) practice management guidelines work group: update to practice management guidelines for prophylactic antibiotic use in open fractures. J Trauma 2011;70:751–4.

35. Baxter CR. Fluid volume and electrolyte changes in the early post-burn period. Clin Plast Surg 1974;1:693–703.

36. Cancio LC. Initial assessment and fluid resuscitation of burn patients. Surg Clin North Am 2014;94:741–54.

37. Markell KW, Renz EM, White CE, et al. Abdominal complications after severe burns. J Am Coll Surg 2009;208:940–7 [discussion: 7–9].

38. Pham TN, Cancio LC, Gibran NS, et al. American Burn Association practice guidelines burn shock resuscitation. J Burn Care Res 2008;29:257–66.

39. Young DA, Wesson DE. Trauma. In: Cote CJ, Lerman J, Anderson BJ, editors. A practice of anesthesia for infants and children. Philadelphia: Churchill Livingstone Eleesevier; 2018. p. 891–907.

40. Avraham JB, Bhandari M, Frangos SG, et al. Epidemiology of paediatric trauma presenting to US emergency departments: 2006-2012. Inj Prev 2017. [Epub ahead of print].

41. Sauber-Schatz EK, Thomas AM, Cook LJ, Centers for Disease Control and Prevention (CDC). Motor vehicle crashes, medical outcomes, and hospital charges among children aged 1-12 years - crash outcome data evaluation system, 11 states, 2005-2008. MMWR Surveill Summ 2015;64:1–32.

42. Kim PT, Falcone RA Jr. Nonaccidental trauma in pediatric surgery. Surg Clin North Am 2017;97:21–33.

43. Tiyyagura G, Beucher M, Bechtel K. Nonaccidental injury in pediatric patients: detection, evaluation, and treatment. Pediatr Emerg Med Pract 2017;14:1–32.

44. FastStats: life stages and populations, deaths, life expectancy. 2018. Available at: https://www.cdc.gov/nchs/fastats/life-expectancy.htm. Accessed May 12, 2018.

45. Newsroom, news releases, press releases, tip sheet statements, 2017; The Nation's Older Population Is Still Growing. 2017. Available at: https://www.census.gov/newsroom/press-releases/2017/cb17-100.html. Accessed May 12, 2018.

46. Brooks SE, Peetz AB. Evidence-based care of geriatric trauma patients. Surg Clin North Am 2017;97:1157–74.

47. Hruska K, Ruge T. The tragically hip: trauma in elderly patients. Emerg Med Clin North Am 2018;36:219–35.

48. Joyce MF, Gupta A, Azocar RJ. Acute trauma and multiple injuries in the elderly population. Curr Opin Anaesthesiol 2015;28:145–50.

49. Adams SD, Holcomb JD. Geriatric trauma. Curr Opin Crit Care 2015;21:520–6.

50. Huls CK, Detlefs C. Trauma in pregnancy. Semin Perinatol 2018;42:13–20.

51. Mendez-Figueroa H, Dahlke JD, Vrees RA, et al. Trauma in pregnancy: an updated systematic review. Am J Obstet Gynecol 2013;209:1–10.

52. Jain V, Chari R, Maslovitz S, et al. Guidelines for the management of a pregnant trauma patient. J Obstet Gynaecol Can 2015;37:553–74.

53. Battaloglu E, McDonnell D, Chu J, et al. Epidemiology and outcomes of pregnancy and obstetric complications in trauma in the United Kingdom. Injury 2016;47:184-7.
54. Onzuka J, Worster A, McCreadie B. Is computerized tomography of trauma patients associated with a transfer delay to a regional trauma centre? CJEM 2008;10:205-8.
55. Quick JA, Bartels AN, Coughenour JP, et al. Trauma transfers and definitive imaging: patient benefit but at what cost? Am Surg 2013;79:301-4.
56. Jones AC, Woldemikael D, Fisher T, et al. Repeated computed tomographic scans in transferred trauma patients: Indications, costs, and radiation exposure. J Trauma Acute Care Surg 2012;73:1564-9.

Trauma Airway Management

Induction Agents, Rapid Versus Slower Sequence Intubations, and Special Considerations

Stephen R. Estime, MD[a],*, Catherine M. Kuza, MD[b]

KEYWORDS

- Trauma airway • Trauma airway management • Slow-sequence intubation
- Trauma anesthesia • Trauma anesthesiology • Cervical spine injury
- Trauma induction • Trauma intubation

KEY POINTS

- Using an induction agent with a favorable hemodynamic profile is important in trauma airway management because these patients are at high risk for cardiovascular collapse.
- Rapid-sequence induction and intubation is the most common technique in the trauma patient and quickly provides intubating conditions that can minimize aspiration risk, but poses other risks in some patients.
- "Slow-sequence" induction and intubation may be preferable in trauma patients at risk for failed intubation and cardiovascular collapse.
- Cervical spine instability, anatomic disruptions, bleeding, and combativeness in trauma patients complicate intubation so developing preemptive strategies addressing these crises can improve airway management success.
- Development and maintenance of skills in a variety of urgent airway management approaches is essential for practicing trauma anesthesiologists.

INTRODUCTION

Trauma airway management is often performed in unfamiliar settings (ie, emergency department [ED], trauma bay, radiology scanner, ambulance), where space is limited, patient risk is high, and time is of the essence.[1] This article focuses on considerations

Both authors have no disclosures to discuss.

[a] Department of Anesthesiology and Critical Care, University of Chicago Medicine, 5841 South Maryland Avenue, MC-4028, Chicago, IL 60637, USA; [b] Department of Anesthesiology and Critical Care, Keck School of Medicine, University of Southern California, 1520 San Pablo Street, Suite 3451, Los Angeles, CA 90033, USA

* Corresponding author. University of Chicago Medicine, 5841 South Maryland Avenue, MC-4028, Chicago, IL 60637.

E-mail addresses: sestime@gmail.com; sestime@dacc.uchicago.edu

Anesthesiology Clin 37 (2019) 33–50
https://doi.org/10.1016/j.anclin.2018.09.002
1932-2275/19/© 2018 Elsevier Inc. All rights reserved.

anesthesiology.theclinics.com

for induction regimens, airway management techniques, and complex airway scenarios in trauma patients.

INDUCTION AGENTS

Induction agents provide sedation; reduce distress, tachycardia, and hypertension; and improve intubating conditions. An ideal agent should have a rapid onset and minimal adverse effects. Titrating induction doses carefully to limit adverse effects is important because these drugs may cause hypotension through myocardial depression and peripheral vasodilation. This effect must be weighed against the risks of inadequate dosing, including poorer intubating conditions, tachycardia, hypertension, pain, and awareness. Awareness is a well-documented complication of trauma and emergency surgery[2–4] and is more likely when hemodynamic decompensation is likely, prompting reduced dosing. Induction agents that achieve their goals with limited side effects are more favorable for this reason.[2] Popular induction agents in trauma include etomidate, ketamine, propofol, and midazolam.[5]

Etomidate is commonly used for its minimal effect on blood pressure. It is an imidazole derivative and potent, short-acting anesthetic. Similar to most sedative induction agents, it is a γ-aminobutyric acid receptor agonist. Hemodynamic stability during etomidate induction occurs via α-adrenoreceptor stimulation.[6,7] Typical intravenous (IV) doses of 0.2 to 0.3 mg/kg achieve induction goals while preserving cardiac output, inotropy, systemic vascular resistance, and arterial pressure. Often minimal dose adjustments are needed even during hypovolemia and hemorrhagic shock.[8] Etomidate causes adrenocortical suppression through 11 β-hydroxylase inhibition for at least 12 to 48 hours, even when administered as a single dose, which has led some providers to avoid its use in trauma patients.[2,9] Although continuous infusions have been correlated with increased mortality,[10,11] single-dose etomidate has not been associated with increased mortality.[12–17]

Ketamine is also commonly used in trauma because of its limited effect on blood pressure. IV doses of 1 to 2 mg/kg take effect in less than 1 minute and last up to 20 minutes. Ketamine's high lipid solubility and low protein binding allow for rapid blood-brain equilibration and onset.[2] It causes anesthesia and analgesia through N-methyl-D-aspartate antagonism and increases heart rate, contractility, and mean arterial pressure via catecholamine receptor stimulation.[18] Higher doses of ketamine directly reduce cardiac contractility and can precipitate cardiovascular collapse especially in those with catecholamine depletion.[2,5,18,19] Ketamine preserves respiratory drive, but increases respiratory secretions.[20,21] Ketamine may increase intracranial pressure (ICP), and its administration in patients with elevated ICP is controversial.[2,22,23] A more detailed discussion is provided later. Comparisons between etomidate and ketamine for use during rapid-sequence intubation (RSI) have not found differences in mortality.[24]

Unlike etomidate and ketamine, propofol has a pronounced hypotensive effect and is best reserved for hemodynamically stable, euvolemic patients. The potency of propofol increases with the severity of shock[25] so slower, titrated dosing in combination with vasopressors (eg, phenylephrine) is required in hemodynamically unstable patients.

Benzodiazepines cause sedation and amnesia. Midazolam is the most rapidly acting benzodiazepine, but the recommended induction dose of 0.2 mg/kg may cause hypotension and significant dose reduction is required in hemodynamically unstable patients.[18,26] Such dose reductions reduce onset of action and may increase awareness.[2,27] Barbiturates, such as thiopental and methohexital, are less commonly used. These agents reduce ICP, inotropy, baroreceptor responsiveness, and arterial vascular tone, potentially worsening hemodynamic instability.[2]

NEUROMUSCULAR BLOCKING AGENTS

Neuromuscular blocking agents (NMBAs) can improve success and reduce complications in emergency intubations.[28–30] Succinylcholine and rocuronium are the most commonly used agents in trauma. A 1.5 to 2 mg/kg IV dose of succinylcholine acts within 30 seconds by depolarizing postsynaptic neuromuscular junction receptors causing receptor desensitization and inactivation.[19,31] In most cases hydrolysis by plasma cholinesterase causes neuromuscular function to return within 10 minutes, although the duration of succinylcholine may vary widely in critically ill patients.[32] Succinylcholine may increase intraocular pressure and ICP.[33] Although anecdotes have been described, published case reports of succinylcholine-induced eye damage are extremely rare.[31,34] Succinylcholine is also a trigger for malignant hyperthermia and may induce hyperkalemia (as seen with stroke, neuromuscular disease, burns, rhabdomyolysis, and so forth).[18,31]

Rocuronium induces muscle relaxation by antagonizing post-synaptic neuromuscular junction receptors. Although the normal dose of 0.6 mg/kg produces adequate intubating conditions in 2 to 3 minutes, doubling the dose reduces peak onset time to approximately 1 minute.[18] Rocuronium has minimal side effects, although its longer duration could be problematic in a "cannot mask, cannot intubate" scenario. Sugammadex was recently introduced to the United States and can quickly reverse rocuronium-induced neuromuscular blockade. Sugammadex has greatly facilitated the use of rocuronium in trauma intubation.

GENERAL CONSIDERATIONS IN TRAUMA AIRWAY MANAGEMENT
Difficult Airway Prediction

Risk factors for difficult mask ventilation and intubation should be identified early so primary and backup airway plans are established. ROMAN and LEMON are prospectively validated mnemonics identifying factors for difficult ventilation and intubation, respectively (**Table 1**).[35,36] If time permits, documentation of previous airway management episodes should be reviewed, especially when a difficult airway is suspected. Understanding the mechanism of injury can help guide the evaluation of the injured airway. Specific trauma-induced airway alterations are discussed in more detail later.

Patient Compliance

Behavioral noncompliance and combativeness are common in trauma and can impact the feasibility of awake or lightly sedated intubations. Alternatively, a hypoactive,

Table 1	
Mnemonics for difficult mask ventilation and intubation	
Difficult Mask Ventilation (ROMAN)[35]	**Difficult Intubation (LEMON)[36]**
Radiation (head and neck)/Restriction (lung)	Look externally
Obesity/Obstruction/Obstructive sleep apnea	Evaluate 3-3-2 rule[a]
Mask seal/Mallampati/Male	Mallampati score
Age >55	Obstruction/Obesity
No teeth	Neck mobility

[a] 3-3-2 rule: three finger breadths interincisor distance, three finger breadths hyoid-mental distance, and two finger breaths thyroid notch to floor of mouth distance.

comatose patient may require little, if any, induction agent to facilitate intubation. Determining an airway plan based on anticipated compliance can help avoid failed airway attempts and limit doses of induction agents when appropriate.

Hemodynamic Stability

Hemodynamic instability is common in trauma from damage to vital organs, sympathetic surges, bleeding, and inflammation. Furthermore, patients initially appearing stable can rapidly deteriorate on induction. Induction agents cause myocardial depression and sympathetic attenuation to varying degrees. Fluid and blood product resuscitation, pneumothorax decompression, vasopressor therapy, and correcting metabolic abnormalities can attenuate the hemodynamic effects of induction and intubation.

Gastric Aspiration

Trauma-induced physiologic changes may result in delayed gastric emptying, which can then increase the risk of aspiration.[37] Administering drugs to neutralize acid production and/or performing gastric decompression are helpful but often not feasible in trauma. RSI may reduce aspiration, but must be weighed against the risk of a failed airway.[38,39] In cooperative patients with an anticipated difficult airway, an awake intubation can preserve protective airway reflexes and hemodynamic status. Although RSI is the most common airway management approach in trauma, understanding when to use an alternative airway technique is challenging.[40]

STRATEGIES FOR AIRWAY MANAGEMENT: RAPID-SEQUENCE INTUBATION, "SLOWER-SEQUENCE" INTUBATION, AND AWAKE INTUBATIONS

RSI is commonly performed in trauma intubations by applying cricoid pressure (controversial), followed by an induction agent and NMBA in rapid succession without mask ventilation.[31,41] RSI is used in up to 85% of trauma/emergency intubations,[38,39,42–44] because it is the fastest intubation technique and may reduce aspiration. Fixed, predetermined dosing may be associated with overdosing and underdosing complications, namely awareness and hemodynamic instability. In practice, modifications to the RSI technique are often required.

Slower-sequence intubation (SSI) involves the slow titration of induction agents. It may be done in an anticipated difficult airway, intolerance to preoxygenation, hemodynamic instability, or to ensure unconsciousness before giving an NMBA.[45] It may be used in combination with physiologic optimization through aggressive preoxygenation, gastric decompression, and titration of vasopressors.[40,45] With prolonged induction times, aspiration is a serious risk.[31] No data exist that compare RSI with SSI on the effects of aspiration, hemodynamic stability, or awareness.[31]

An "awake" intubation implies that patients are awake and aware of the intubation process (**Fig. 1**). It is normally performed in spontaneously breathing patients, and facilitated with application of topical local anesthetic. An awake intubation requires more time, expertise, and patient compliance and is not always feasible in trauma patients. Occasionally a lightly sedated approach is needed to facilitate intubation. Ketamine is a popular choice because airway patency and respiratory drive are better preserved.

The airway plan should factor in patient injuries, comorbidities, mental status, risk of difficult intubation/ventilation, hemodynamic status, aspiration risk, available equipment, and provider experience and skills. Factoring the anticipated risk of each should allow for a more flexible, thoughtful airway plan that better avoids adverse events.

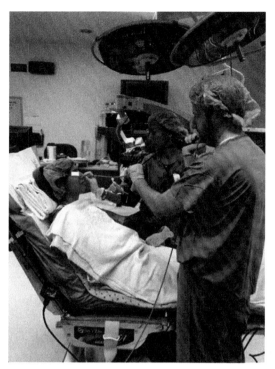

Fig. 1. Awake fiberoptic intubation–fiberoptic laryngoscopy. (*From* Linkov G, Soliman AMS. Infections and edema. Anesthesiology Clin 2015;33(2):334; with permission.)

SPECIAL CONSIDERATIONS
Cervical Spine Injuries

Cervical spine (C-spine) injury occurs in up to 5% of trauma patients, of which 14% are unstable.[46] Early intubation is recommended in C-spine injuries associated with respiratory distress,[47] such as those with spinal injuries above C5 where diaphragmatic dysfunction and paralysis are common.[48] C-spine injuries may be associated with edema and cervical hematomas, which can cause airway obstruction[49] and make intubations more challenging.[50] Airway management with C-spine precaution is best accomplished by removing the anterior portion of the cervical collar and performing manual in-line stabilization (MILS) of the neck to minimize further injury from excessive cervical motion.[47,51–53] Application of cricoid pressure during RSI may impede the ability to intubate.[46,54–58] All intubation maneuvers produce some level of C-spine mobility, but jaw thrust or bag mask ventilation produce more movement than direct laryngoscopy (DL) (**Fig. 2**).[54] Currently, orotracheal intubation is recommended.[46,47,57]

The American Society of Anesthesiology (ASA) Committee on Trauma and Emergency Preparedness has modified their difficult airway algorithm for trauma patients, and provided specific recommendations for C-spine injury (**Fig. 3**).[57]

The use of video laryngoscopy (VL) in C-spine injuries has increased among providers[52,58–60]; however, evidence for its superiority over DL is lacking.[57,61] VL does not produce less C-spine mobility than DL.[52,54,59,61] VL is associated with an improved glottic view compared with DL,[47,59] and may decrease the number of intubation attempts.[62,63] However, overall intubation success rates with VL and DL are similar.[59]

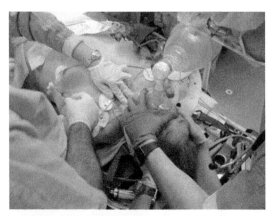

Fig. 2. Emergency intubation of a trauma patient, immobilized on a long spine board. The front of the cervical collar is removed once in-line manual stabilization of the spine is established, allowing for cricoid pressure and greater excursion of the mandible. (*From* Dutton RP. Spinal cord injury. Int Anesthesiol Clin 2002;40:111; with permission.)

In particularly difficult airways, a fiberoptic bronchoscopy (FIOB) may be required.[55] FIOB intubations are associated with the least C-spine movement,[54,56,64–66] although secretions and blood may obstruct views.[54,56,67] Additionally, FIOB is time consuming when performed awake because it requires cooperation and time for local anesthetic topicalization. In emergent situations, an asleep DL with MILS may be the most rapid way to secure an airway.[54,61,64] In difficult airway management, the addition of a gum elastic bougie during DL may reduce intubating times and increase success rates.[46,68] Laryngeal mask airways (LMAs) may be used as a temporizing adjunct during a failed airway or difficult mask ventilation.[46,56] However, LMAs can exert significant pressure on the posterior airway and cause cervical vertebrae displacement in unstable C-spine injuries.[56,64] Rescue LMA may be safer than returning to bag mask ventilation with jaw thrust, because it is associated with less C-spine movement, but there are insufficient studies in a difficult airway scenario specifically in patients with C-spine injury to provide definitive recommendations.

Ultimately, the airway approach should be selected based on the providers' experience, available equipment/resources, patients' injuries, airway difficulty, aspiration risk, and patient cooperation.[52,54,55,67,69]

Facial Trauma

Facial trauma from blunt or penetrating injuries may increase the difficulty of intubation and bag-mask ventilation because of nasopharyngeal and oropharyngeal edema, bleeding, airway obstruction, and jaw dysfunction.[70–72] Displaced condylar fractures may result in limited mouth opening and trismus may occur with mandibular and zygomatic arch injuries.[72,73] When blood pools in the oropharynx or is swallowed in large amounts, the gag reflex may be triggered and the risks of aspiration and regurgitation are increased.[72,73]

Blunt facial trauma may result in specific fracture patterns known as Le Fort fractures (I-III) **(Fig. 4)**.[74] Le Fort II and III fractures may be associated with basal skull fractures, cerebrospinal fluid rhinorrhea, and ophthalmic complications.[72,74] Facial trauma classification can also be divided into facial thirds (upper, middle, and lower) **(Fig. 5)**. The middle-third region is most commonly injured.[75,76] Up to 10% of facial fractures

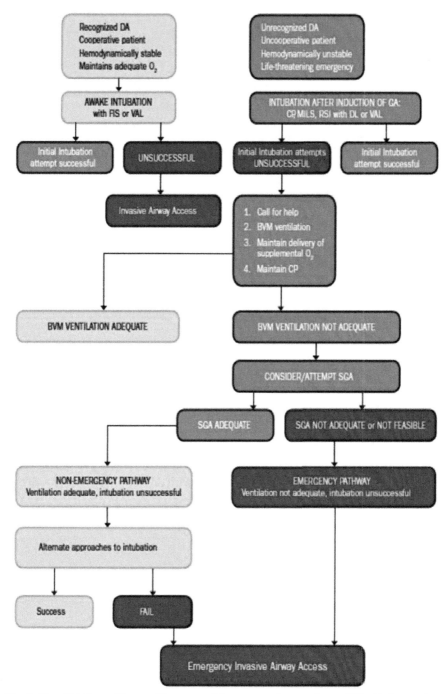

Fig. 3. The ASA Committee on Trauma and Emergency Preparedness difficult airway algorithm for trauma patients. BVM, bag-valve-mask; CP, cricoid pressure; DA, difficult airway; RS, rigid scope; SGA, supraglottic airway; VAL, video-assisted laryngoscopy. (*From* Hagberg CA, Kaslow O. Difficult airway management algorithm in trauma updated by COTEP. ASA Monitor 2014;78(9):59; with permission.)

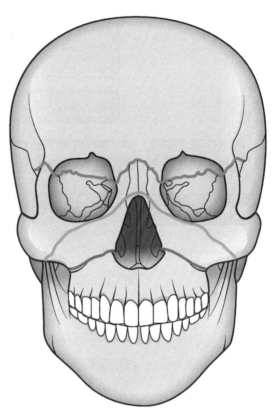

Fig. 4. Le Fort fractures I-III (*pink line* = Le Fort I; *green line* = Le Fort II; *blue line* = Le Fort III). (*Courtesy of* C.M. Kuza, MD, Los Angeles, CA.)

have associated C-spine injuries.[70–72,74] In patients with maxillofacial injuries, six specific scenarios may complicate airway management (**Box 1**).[70,72,73]

Anesthesiologists and surgeons should work together in securing the airway in patients with maxillofacial trauma.[71] In stable and cooperative patients, awake FIOB is reasonable[73,77] but may not be feasible because of blood, vomitus, and secretions. If awake intubation fails, an awake tracheostomy under local anesthesia may be the next best step.[57] Nasal instrumentation or intubation should be avoided in basilar skull and nasal fractures to prevent intracranial tube placement and cranial vault damage.[71,72] Blind intubations are not recommended because they may dislodge foreign bodies and cause airway obstruction, or create a false lumen.[71] Nasal intubation using FIOB is reasonable if the fracture does not cross midline and there is no damage to the cribriform plate on computed tomography imaging.[72] When time is limited, any intubating technique (eg, DL, VL) may be considered based on provider preference.[77] An RSI with DL may be the most efficient way to secure an airway emergently in patients with facial fractures. An approach to airway management in maxillofacial trauma is demonstrated in **Fig. 6**.

Submental intubation
Submental intubations are performed when a clear intraoral field is required, nasal intubation is contraindicated, and the patient does not need to remain intubated

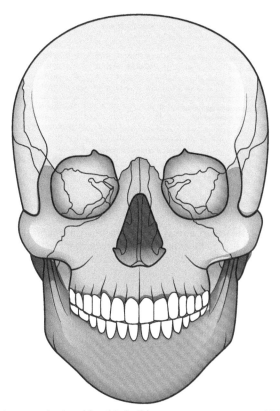

Fig. 5. Facial fractures as depicted by thirds (*blue* = upper; *green* = middle; *pink* = lower third). (*Courtesy of* C.M. Kuza, MD, Los Angeles, CA.)

postoperatively.[77] An existing oral endotracheal tube is easily converted to a submental position, by tunneling the tube through the mouth floor via an incision between the mandibular angle and the chin (**Fig. 7**).[57,70] It allows for dental occlusion, produces minimal soft tissue distortion, and motor and sensory damage is unlikely.[77] It may

---

Box 1
Scenarios associated with maxillofacial injuries complicating airway management

Displaced maxillary fracture obstructing nasopharyngeal airway

Bilateral mandibular fractures resulting in posterior tongue displacement and airway obstruction when supine

Secretions, blood, teeth, bone fragments, and so forth causing airway obstruction at various locations in the respiratory tract

Severe hemorrhage resulting in obstruction

Airway edema from head/neck injuries

Neck injuries causing laryngotracheal distortion/edema causing cervical airway compromise

Data from Refs.[70,72,73]

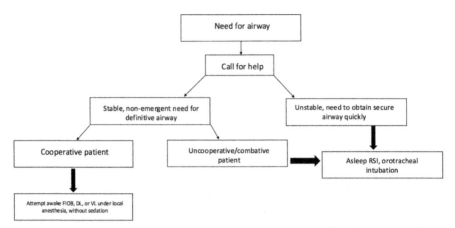

Fig. 6. A suggested approach to airway management in maxillofacial trauma. (*Adapted from* Mercer SJ, Jones CP, Bridge M, et al. Systematic review of the anaesthetic management of non-iatrogenic acute adult airway trauma. Br J Anaesth 2016;117 Suppl 1:i55; with permission.)

be associated with damage to the endotracheal tube, difficulty suctioning, and increased airway pressure.[77] Submental intubation is contraindicated in patients who require postoperative ventilator support[70,77] or have comminuted mandibular fractures.[70] Complications include bleeding, damage to lingual and mandibular

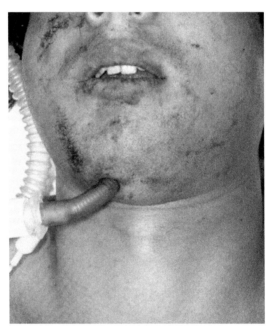

Fig. 7. In a submental approach for intubation, an endotracheal tube is inserted through an incision between the mandibular angle and the chin into the floor of the mouth. (*From* Lima Júnior SM, Asprino L, Fernandes Moreira RW, et al. A retrospective analysis of submental intubation in maxillofacial trauma patients. J Oral Maxillofac Surg 2011;69(7):2003; with permission.)

branch of the facial nerves, damage to sublingual and submandibular glands, desaturation, accidental extubation, endobronchial intubation, local infection, fistula, or scarring.[70,77] A spiral reinforced flexometallic endotracheal tube is preferred to prevent tube kinking.[70,77]

Surgical airway

A tracheostomy may be performed in maxillofacial injuries with airway compromise with or without previous failed intubation attempts. It is especially useful in patients requiring prolonged mechanical ventilation.[71] Tracheostomy is associated with numerous complications including: bleeding, recurrent laryngeal nerve damage, subcutaneous emphysema, and tracheal stenosis.[77] In emergent conditions, a cricothyrotomy may be faster and associated with fewer complications.[71]

Laryngotracheal Injuries

The incidence of laryngotracheal injuries in the United States is less than 0.05%.[78] Signs that suggest the presence of laryngotracheal injury include: neck trauma, stridor, subcutaneous emphysema, crepitus, hoarseness, dysphonia, aphonia, dyspnea, dysphagia, neck or throat pain, large-volume hemoptysis, presence of neurologic deficits, tracheal deviation, neck hematoma/lacerations/contusions, and/or wound bubbling.[72,78,79] These injuries can occur from penetrating and blunt force neck trauma.[80,81] Injuries from blunt trauma are most commonly the result of motor vehicle accidents (59%) and crush injuries (27%).[80] About 30% of patients with penetrating neck injuries have aerodigestive injuries, and associated vascular injuries are also common.[79] Laryngotracheal injuries are more common than pharyngoesophageal injuries, but both are associated with mortality rates of approximately 20%.[79] In patients with laryngotracheal injuries, intubation should be performed under direct visualization to prevent creation of a false lumen or inducing a tracheal transection.[79] Awake FIOB is preferred to prevent losing a patent airway in a spontaneously breathing patient. *Cricoid pressure should be avoided because it can exacerbate injury*.[78–80,82] A surgical airway may be necessary when extensive maxillofacial trauma, severe upper airway distortion, or known airway edema is present. Cricothyrotomy is often preferred[79] for its ease, efficiency, and few complications.[80] Patients with complete tracheal transection typically die at the scene and those who make it to the hospital have high mortality rates.[80] During a complete tracheal transection, the lower end of the trachea may be pulled up with forceps through the wound, and an endotracheal tube may be placed into the lower trachea before heading to the operating room for definitive management.[80] Tracheotomy is recommended in partial or complete transection of the trachea or larynx, extensive laryngeal fractures causing skeletal breakdown, profound disruption of airway anatomy, and/or anterior neck hematoma.[79,80]

Suspected Difficult Airway/Difficult Intubation

The risk of a difficult airway is increased in urgent and emergent settings.[69] If possible, trauma patients should be carefully examined to identify risks for difficult ventilation/intubation.[47] The ASA Committee on Trauma and Emergency Preparedness created a modified difficult airway algorithm for trauma patients (see **Fig. 3**). The trauma difficult airway algorithm differs from the 2013 ASA algorithm in acknowledging that preassessment of the airway may not be possible and that a surgical airway may be the best initial airway option. The ASA algorithm also recognizes that waking up the patient after induction may not be possible, and that cricoid pressure and MILS may be abandoned if they hinder securing the airway. VL has been increasingly used in trauma patients and has comparable outcomes to DL. Trauma airway management is best addressed using a team-based approach. Experienced airway providers and those who can perform surgical airways should be present. Additional providers to perform MILS and administer cricoid pressure are often valuable. Finally, a plan for failed or difficult airway management should be defined when performing intubations in trauma patients.

Massive Pulmonary Hemorrhage/Hemoptysis

Massive hemoptysis may result from blunt or penetrating trauma. In hemodynamically stable patients, computed tomography angiography is the preferred diagnostic test.[83] In unstable patients without control of pulmonary hemorrhage, mortality rates exceed 50%.[83] Bright red blood in the mouth on airway examination should prompt an oropharyngeal examination to identify the bleeding sources. Bleeding from deeper structures, such as central pulmonary vessels, can cause alveolar flooding, parenchymal damage, hypoxemia, and intrapulmonary shunting.[84] Such cases may present as hemothorax and should be suspected in cases of massive hemothorax when the patient is in shock, has hypoxia, and has absent breath sounds on auscultation.[51]

Intubation with a large-diameter endotracheal tube should be performed if pulmonary hemorrhage is suspected.[85] Flexible bronchoscopy can help determine the site of the bleed, although severe bleeding may make vision difficult and suction capability is limited.[85] Rigid bronchoscopy may be a useful alternative to control the bleeding, especially if the source is in a proximal airway.[85] If the source is identified, the patient should be placed with the bleeding side down to avoid blood flow into the uninvolved lung. Lung isolation may be performed by advancing the single-lumen tube into the unaffected bronchus under bronchoscopic guidance, bronchial blocker isolation, or by placement of a double-lumen tube. A tamponading balloon catheter, hemostatic topical agents, and cautery may be used to treat bleeding.[85] The evidence for IV tranexamic acid[86] and IV factor VIIa[87] is limited. Emergent thoracotomy is a last-line therapy and is associated with high morbidity and mortality.[51,85]

The Combative Patient

Trauma patients can present with coexisting intoxication, psychiatric illness, infection, pain, hypoxemia, hypoperfusion, language barriers, and traumatic brain injuries (TBIs).[73,88] A review of trauma patients intubated early in the ED revealed that 85% were intubated for altered mental status or combativeness. More than 50% of these patients had a significant TBI,[89] which is a risk factor for agitation.[88,90] Early intubation may facilitate work-up, imaging, treatment, and prevention of self-inflicted injury.[47,73,88]

Guidelines to manage agitation in trauma patients are limited. Pharmacologic interventions are associated with worsened mental status, respiratory depression, and hemodynamic instability, and can mask symptoms of life-threatening injuries.[91] In the combative patient, "awake" airway management options are challenging and sedated or asleep intubations may be required. Ketamine may be advantageous because it can be administered intramuscularly while preserving hemodynamics and respiratory drive in patients with an anticipated difficult airway and/or hemodynamic instability.

Traumatic Brain Injury and Increased Intracranial Pressure

TBIs represent most trauma presenting to the ED.[51] Intubation may be required in those presenting with a Glasgow Coma Score less than or equal to 8 because such patients may not be able to protect their airway. Coexisting C-spine injuries are common and precautions should be taken.[60] Avoiding hypoxemia by preoxygenation and maximizing first-pass intubation success is important because desaturation may adversely affect neurologic outcomes in TBI.[92–94] RSI is recommended and, should initial attempts at intubation fail, quickly progressing toward a surgical airway is important to minimize hypoxemia.

In such patients the ICP may be elevated and prophylactic head of the bed elevation to approximately 30° attenuates ICP elevations during intubation.[93] Giving induction agents before airway instrumentation blunts sympathetic responses that may otherwise elevate ICP, worsen edema or hematoma expansion, and may precipitate brainstem herniation.[92–94] Opioids, lidocaine, and β-blockers[93] are used as adjuncts to further blunt sympathetic responses to instrumentation. VL may also reduce sympathetic response compared with DL.[92,94] Although blunting sympathetic responses to instrumentation is important, it should not be at the expense of hemodynamic collapse. Etomidate and ketamine may be reasonable choices in hemodynamically unstable patients.[18,60,93] Although ketamine may increase ICP, the significance is controversial and ketamine use has not been associated with worse neurologic outcomes in TBI.[22,60,95]

SUMMARY

Airway management in trauma patients is uniquely challenging. Standardized guidelines are limited and the technique and induction regimen should be individualized. Although providers may choose plans with which they are most comfortable, recognizing risk factors that influence airway management is an important aspect in developing a flexible approach. Plans that involve awake or lightly sedated patients during SSI may be required and identifying patients that best benefit from these approaches may improve outcomes in trauma patients. It is hoped that future work identifying airway approaches, induction dosing, and risk factors that may alter traditional plans will improve the care of trauma patients.

REFERENCES

1. Crewdson K, Nolan J. Management of the trauma airway. Trauma 2011;13(3): 221–32.
2. Morris C, Perris A, Klein J, et al. Anaesthesia in haemodynamically compromised emergency patients: does ketamine represent the best choice of induction agent? Anaesthesia 2009;64(5):532–9.
3. Ranta SO-V, Laurila R, Saario J, et al. Awareness with recall during general anesthesia: incidence and risk factors. Anesth Analg 1998;86(5):1084–9.
4. Bogetz MS, Katz JA. Recall of surgery for major trauma. Anesthesiology 1984; 61(1):6–9.
5. Groth CM, Acquisto NM, Khadem T. Current practices and safety of medication use during rapid sequence intubation. J Crit Care 2018;45:65–70.
6. Bergen JM, Smith DC. A review of etomidate for rapid sequence intubation in the emergency department. J Emerg Med 1997;15(2):221–30.
7. Pascoe PJ, Ilkiw JE, Haskins SC, et al. Cardiopulmonary effects of etomidate in hypovolemic dogs. Am J Vet Res 1992;53(11):2178–82.
8. Johnson KB, Egan TD, Layman J, et al. The influence of hemorrhagic shock on etomidate: a pharmacokinetic and pharmacodynamic analysis. Anesth Analg 2003;96(5):1360–8. Table of contents.
9. Vinclair M, Broux C, Faure P, et al. Duration of adrenal inhibition following a single dose of etomidate in critically ill patients. Intensive Care Med 2008;34(4):714–9.
10. Ledingham I. Influence of sedation on mortality in critically ill multiple trauma patients. Lancet 1983;321(8336):1270.

11. Watt I, Ledingham IM. Mortality amongst multiple trauma patients admitted to an intensive therapy unit. Anaesthesia 1984;39(10):973–81.
12. Hinkewich C, Green R. The impact of etomidate on mortality in trauma patients. Can J Anaesth 2014;61(7):650–5.
13. Banh KV, James S, Hendey GW, et al. Single-dose etomidate for intubation in the trauma patient. J Emerg Med 2012;43(5):e277–82.
14. Tekwani KL, Watts HF, Rzechula KH, et al. A prospective observational study of the effect of etomidate on septic patient mortality and length of stay. Acad Emerg Med 2009;16(1):11–4.
15. Bruder EA, Ball IM, Ridi S, et al. Single induction dose of etomidate versus other induction agents for endotracheal intubation in critically ill patients. Cochrane Database Syst Rev 2015;(1):CD010225.
16. McPhee LC, Badawi O, Fraser GL, et al. Single-dose etomidate is not associated with increased mortality in ICU patients with sepsis: analysis of a large electronic ICU database. Crit Care Med 2013;41(3):774–83.
17. Dmello D, Taylor S, O'Brien J, et al. Outcomes of etomidate in severe sepsis and septic shock. Chest 2010;138(6):1327–32.
18. Butterworth JF, Mackey DC, Wasnick JD, et al. Morgan & Mikhail's clinical anesthesiology [Chapters: 9–11]. New York: McGraw-Hill; 2013.
19. [Chapters: 30, 34]. In: Miller RD, editor. Miller's anesthesia. 8th edition. Philadelphia: Elsevier/Saunders; 2015.
20. Himmelseher S, Durieux ME. Revising a dogma: ketamine for patients with neurological injury? Anesth Analg 2005;101(2):524–34. Table of contents.
21. Berkenbosch JW, Graff GR, Stark JM. Safety and efficacy of ketamine sedation for infant flexible fiberoptic bronchoscopy. Chest 2004;125(3):1132–7.
22. Cohen L, Athaide V, Wickham ME, et al. The effect of ketamine on intracranial and cerebral perfusion pressure and health outcomes: a systematic review. Ann Emerg Med 2015;65(1):43–51.e2.
23. Albanèse J, Arnaud S, Rey M, et al. Ketamine decreases intracranial pressure and electroencephalographic activity in traumatic brain injury patients during propofol sedation. Anesthesiology 1997;87(6):1328–34.
24. Jabre P, Combes X, Ricard-Hibon A, et al. Etomidate versus ketamine for rapid sequence intubation in acutely ill patients: a multicenter randomized controlled trial. Crit Care 2009;13(Suppl 1):P405.
25. Shafer SL. Shock values. Anesthesiology 2004;101(3):567–8.
26. Sagarin MJ, Barton ED, Sakles JC, et al. Underdosing of midazolam in emergency endotracheal intubation. Acad Emerg Med 2003;10(4):329–38.
27. White PF. Comparative evaluation of intravenous agents for rapid sequence induction: thiopental, ketamine, and midazolam. Anesthesiology 1982;57(4):279–84.
28. Bozeman WP, Kleiner DM, Huggett V. A comparison of rapid-sequence intubation and etomidate-only intubation in the prehospital air medical setting. Prehosp Emerg Care 2006;10(1):8–13.
29. Wilcox SR, Bittner EA, Elmer J, et al. Neuromuscular blocking agent administration for emergent tracheal intubation is associated with decreased prevalence of procedure-related complications. Crit Care Med 2012;40(6):1808–13.
30. Lundstrøm LH, Duez CH, Nørskov AK, et al. Avoidance versus use of neuromuscular blocking agents for improving conditions during tracheal intubation or direct laryngoscopy in adults and adolescents. Cochrane Database Syst Rev 2017;(5):CD009237.

31. El-Orbany M, Connolly LA. Rapid sequence induction and intubation: current controversy. Anesth Analg 2010;110(5):1318–25.
32. Dell-Kuster S, Levano S, Burkhart CS, et al. Predictors of the variability in neuro-muscular block duration following succinylcholine: a prospective, observational study. Eur J Anaesthesiol 2015;32(10):687–96.
33. Kelly RE, Dinner M, Turner LS, et al. Succinylcholine increases intraocular pressure in the human eye with the extraocular muscles detached. Anesthesiology 1993;79(5):948–52.
34. Vachon CA, Warner DO, Bacon DR. Succinylcholine and the open globe. Tracing the teaching. Anesthesiology 2003;99(1):220–3.
35. Reed MJ, Dunn MJG, McKeown DW. Can an airway assessment score predict difficulty at intubation in the emergency department? Emerg Med J 2005;22(2):99–102.
36. Walls RM, Murphy MF, editors. Manual of emergency airway management. 4th edition. Philadelphia: Wolters Kluwer/Lippincott Williams & Wilkins Heath; 2012.
37. Robinson M, Davidson A. Aspiration under anaesthesia: risk assessment and decision-making. Cont Educ Anaesth Crit Care Pain 2014;14(4):171–5.
38. Sakles JC, Laurin EG, Rantapaa AA, et al. Airway management in the emergency department: a one-year study of 610 tracheal intubations. Ann Emerg Med 1998;31(3):325–32.
39. Li J, Murphy-Lavoie H, Bugas C, et al. Complications of emergency intubation with and without paralysis. Am J Emerg Med 1999;17(2):141–3.
40. Mosier JM, Joshi R, Hypes C, et al. The physiologically difficult airway. West J Emerg Med 2015;16(7):1109–17.
41. Koerber JP, Roberts GEW, Whitaker R, et al. Variation in rapid sequence induction techniques: current practice in Wales. Anaesthesia 2009;64(1):54–9.
42. Sagarin MJ, Barton ED, Chng Y-M, et al, National Emergency Airway Registry Investigators. Airway management by US and Canadian emergency medicine residents: a multicenter analysis of more than 6,000 endotracheal intubation attempts. Ann Emerg Med 2005;46(4):328–36.
43. Bair AE, Filbin MR, Kulkarni RG, et al. The failed intubation attempt in the emergency department: analysis of prevalence, rescue techniques, and personnel. J Emerg Med 2002;23(2):131–40.
44. Brown CA, Bair AE, Pallin DJ, et al, NEAR III Investigators. Techniques, success, and adverse events of emergency department adult intubations. Ann Emerg Med 2015;65(4):363–70.e1.
45. Weingart SD, Trueger NS, Wong N, et al. Delayed sequence intubation: a prospective observational study. Ann Emerg Med 2015;65(4):349–55.
46. Ollerton JE, Parr MJA, Harrison K, et al. Potential cervical spine injury and difficult airway management for emergency intubation of trauma adults in the emergency department: a systematic review. Emerg Med J 2006;23(1):3–11.
47. Mayglothling J, Duane TM, Gibbs M, et al. Emergency tracheal intubation immediately following traumatic injury: an Eastern Association for the Surgery of Trauma practice management guideline. J Trauma Acute Care Surg 2012;73(5 Suppl 4):S333–40.
48. Heath KJ. The effect of laryngoscopy of different cervical spine immobilisation techniques. Anaesthesia 1994;49(10):843–5.
49. Cleiman P, Nemeth J, Vetere P. A significant cervical spine fracture: think of the airway. J Emerg Med 2012;42(2):e23–5.

50. Ahn H, Singh J, Nathens A, et al. Pre-hospital care management of a potential spinal cord injured patient: a systematic review of the literature and evidence-based guidelines. J Neurotrauma 2011;28(8):1341–61.
51. ATLS Subcommittee, American College of Surgeons' Committee on Trauma, International ATLS Working Group. Advanced trauma life support (ATLS®): the ninth edition. J Trauma Acute Care Surg 2013;74(5):1363–6.
52. McCahon RA, Evans DA, Kerslake RW, et al. Cadaveric study of movement of an unstable atlanto-axial (C1/C2) cervical segment during laryngoscopy and intubation using the Airtraq(®) , Macintosh and McCoy laryngoscopes. Anaesthesia 2015;70(4):452–61.
53. Manoach S, Paladino L. Manual in-line stabilization for acute airway management of suspected cervical spine injury: historical review and current questions. Ann Emerg Med 2007;50(3):236–45.
54. Bao F-P, Zhang H-G, Zhu S-M. Anesthetic considerations for patients with acute cervical spinal cord injury. Neural Regen Res 2017;12(3):499–504.
55. Kuza CM, Vavilala MS, Speck RM, et al. Use of survey and Delphi process to understand trauma anesthesia care practices. Anesth Analg 2018;126(5):1580–7.
56. Farag E. Airway management for cervical spine surgery. Best Pract Res Clin Anaesthesiol 2016;30(1):13–25.
57. Hagberg CA, Kaslow O. Difficult Airway Management Algorithm in Trauma Updated by COTEP. ASA Monitor 2014;78(9):56–60.
58. Diedrich D, Rose P, Brown D. Airway management in cervical spine injury. Curr Anesthesiol Rep 2013;3:197–204.
59. Aziz M. Use of video-assisted intubation devices in the management of patients with trauma. Anesthesiol Clin 2013;31(1):157–66.
60. Jung JY. Airway management of patients with traumatic brain injury/C-spine injury. Korean J Anesthesiol 2015;68(3):213–9.
61. Dooney N, Dagal A. Anesthetic considerations in acute spinal cord trauma. Int J Crit Illn Inj Sci 2011;1(1):36–43.
62. Durga P, Kaur J, Ahmed SY, et al. Comparison of tracheal intubation using the Airtraq(®) and McCoy laryngoscope in the presence of rigid cervical collar simulating cervical immobilisation for traumatic cervical spine injury. Indian J Anaesth 2012;56(6):529–34.
63. Maharaj CH, Buckley E, Harte BH, et al. Endotracheal intubation in patients with cervical spine immobilization: a comparison of Macintosh and Airtraq laryngoscopes. Anesthesiology 2007;107(1):53–9.
64. Ghafoor AU, Martin TW, Gopalakrishnan S, et al. Caring for the patients with cervical spine injuries: what have we learned? J Clin Anesth 2005;17(8):640–9.
65. Bonhomme V, Hartstein G, Hans P. The cervical spine in trauma: implications for the anaesthesiologist. Acta Anaesthesiol Belg 2005;56(4):405–11.
66. Wong DM, Prabhu A, Chakraborty S, et al. Cervical spine motion during flexible bronchoscopy compared with the Lo-Pro GlideScope. Br J Anaesth 2009;102(3):424–30.
67. Holmes MG, Dagal A, Feinstein BA, et al. Airway management practice in adults with an unstable cervical spine: the Harborview Medical Center experience. Anesth Analg 2018. https://doi.org/10.1213/ANE.0000000000003374.
68. Nolan JP, Wilson ME. Orotracheal intubation in patients with potential cervical spine injuries. An indication for the gum elastic bougie. Anaesthesia 1993;48(7):630–3.
69. Martini RP, Larson DM. Clinical evaluation and airway management for adults with cervical spine instability. Anesthesiol Clin 2015;33(2):315–27.

70. Barak M, Bahouth H, Leiser Y, et al. Airway management of the patient with maxillofacial trauma: review of the literature and suggested clinical approach. Biomed Res Int 2015;2015:724032.
71. Coppola S, Froio S, Merli G, et al. Maxillofacial trauma in the emergency department: pearls and pitfalls in airway management. Minerva Anestesiol 2015;81(12):1346–58.
72. Jain U, McCunn M, Smith CE, et al. Management of the traumatized airway. Anesthesiology 2016;124(1):199–206.
73. Kovacs G, Sowers N. Airway management in trauma. Emerg Med Clin North Am 2018;36(1):61–84.
74. Phillips BJ, Turco LM. Le Fort fractures: a collective review. Bull Emerg Trauma 2017;5(4):221–30.
75. Vujcich N, Gebauer D. Current and evolving trends in the management of facial fractures. Aust Dent J 2018;63(Suppl 1):S35–47.
76. Lee K. Global trends in maxillofacial fractures. Craniomaxillofac Trauma Reconstr 2012;5(4):213–22.
77. Gupta B, Prasad A, Ramchandani S, et al. Facing the airway challenges in maxillofacial trauma: a retrospective review of 288 cases at a level I trauma center. Anesth Essays Res 2015;9(1):44–50.
78. Schaefer SD. Management of acute blunt and penetrating external laryngeal trauma. Laryngoscope 2014;124(1):233–44.
79. Nowicki JL, Stew B, Ooi E. Penetrating neck injuries: a guide to evaluation and management. Ann R Coll Surg Engl 2018;100(1):6–11.
80. Raju KNJP, Anandhi D, Surendar R, et al. Blunt trauma neck with complete tracheal transection: a diagnostic and therapeutic challenge to the trauma team. Indian J Crit Care Med 2017;21(6):404–7.
81. Randall DR, Rudmik L, Ball CG, et al. Airway management changes associated with rising radiologic incidence of external laryngotracheal injury. Can J Surg 2018;61(2):121–7.
82. Mercer SJ, Jones CP, Bridge M, et al. Systematic review of the anaesthetic management of non-iatrogenic acute adult airway trauma. Br J Anaesth 2016;117(Suppl 1):i49–59.
83. Khalil A, Fedida B, Parrot A, et al. Severe hemoptysis: from diagnosis to embolization. Diagn Interv Imaging 2015;96(7–8):775–88.
84. Onat S, Ulku R, Avci A, et al. Urgent thoracotomy for penetrating chest trauma: analysis of 158 patients of a single center. Injury 2011;42(9):900–4.
85. Yendamuri S. Massive airway hemorrhage. Thorac Surg Clin 2015;25(3):255–60.
86. Gagnon S, Quigley N, Dutau H, et al. Approach to hemoptysis in the modern era. Can Respir J 2017;2017:1565030.
87. O'Connor JV, Stein DM, Dutton RP, et al. Traumatic hemoptysis treated with recombinant human factor VIIa. Ann Thorac Surg 2006;81(4):1485–7.
88. Garcia A, Yeung LY, Miraflor EJ, et al. Should uncooperative trauma patients with suspected head injury be intubated? Am Surg 2013;79(3):313–20.
89. Sise MJ, Shackford SR, Sise CB, et al. Early intubation in the management of trauma patients: indications and outcomes in 1,000 consecutive patients. J Trauma 2009;66(1):32–9 [discussion: 39–40].
90. Mahmood S, Mahmood O, El-Menyar A, et al. Predisposing factors, clinical assessment, management and outcomes of agitation in the trauma intensive care unit. World J Emerg Med 2018;9(2):105–12.
91. Kuchinski J, Tinkoff G, Rhodes M, et al. Emergency intubation for paralysis of the uncooperative trauma patient. J Emerg Med 1991;9(1–2):9–12.

92. Perkins ZB, Wittenberg MD, Nevin D, et al. The relationship between head injury severity and hemodynamic response to tracheal intubation. J Trauma Acute Care Surg 2013;74(4):1074–80.
93. Bucher J, Koyfman A. Intubation of the neurologically injured patient. J Emerg Med 2015;49(6):920–7.
94. Sharma D, Vavilala MS. Perioperative management of adult traumatic brain injury. Anesthesiol Clin 2012;30(2):333–46.
95. Green SM, Andolfatto G, Krauss BS. Ketamine and intracranial pressure: no contraindication except hydrocephalus. Ann Emerg Med 2015;65(1):52–4.

Viscoelastic Monitoring to Guide the Correction of Perioperative Coagulopathy and Massive Transfusion in Patients with Life-Threatening Hemorrhage

Kevin P. Blaine, MD, MPH[a,b,]*, Marc P. Steurer, MD, MHA, DESA[b,c,1]

KEYWORDS

- Viscoelastic testing • Massive transfusion • Hemostatic resuscitation
- Thromboelastometry • Thromboelastograhy • Hemostasis
- Trauma-induced coagulopathy (TIC) • Acute traumatic coagulopathy (ATC)

KEY POINTS

- Hemostatic resuscitation is critical for massively bleeding patients.
- Conventional laboratory assays of coagulation are insufficient to diagnose acute traumatic coagulopathy.
- Viscoelastic monitoring (VEM) can help the provider to quickly diagnose and monitor coagulopathy in the perioperative setting.
- The interpretation of VEM requires a basic literacy of how the tests are conducted and its basic readouts.
- Used in the right context, VEM can tailor blood component therapies and reduce overuse of empirical transfusions in major trauma patients with intact hemostasis.

INTRODUCTION

Trauma-induced coagulopathy (TIC) develops within the first hour after a major traumatic injury and carries high mortality.[1,2] A cornerstone of hemostatic resuscitation

Disclosure Statement: Both authors have no disclosures, no COI.
a Department of Anesthesiology, Keck School of Medicine of the University of Southern California, 1450 San Pablo Street, HC4 Suite 3600, Los Angeles, CA 90033, USA; b Trauma Anesthesiology Society, Inc, 1001 Fannin St Ste 3700, Houston, TX 77002-6785, USA; c Department of Anesthesia and Perioperative Care, Zuckerberg San Francisco General Hospital and Trauma Center, UCSF School of Medicine, 1001 Potrero Avenue, Building 5, Room 3C-38, San Francisco, CA 94110, USA
1 Senior author.
* Corresponding author.
E-mail address: Kevin.Blaine@med.usc.edu

Anesthesiology Clin 37 (2019) 51–66
https://doi.org/10.1016/j.anclin.2018.09.004
1932-2275/19/© 2018 Elsevier Inc. All rights reserved.
anesthesiology.theclinics.com

is the interruption of pathologic bleeding, including acquired microvascular (coagulopathic) bleeding.[2,3] Point-of-care coagulation testing, including viscoelastic monitoring (VEM) assays such as thromboelastography (TEG) and rotational thromboelastometry (ROTEM), have therefore been welcomed at major trauma centers to help quickly diagnose and monitor TIC. This article reviews the physiologic basis, clinical logic, and evidence base supporting the use of VEM in major trauma.

THE CELL-BASED THEORY OF COAGULATION BEST EXPLAINS HEMOSTASIS

Hemostasis is the process that results in bleeding cessation. The contemporary model of hemostasis is the "Cell-based Theory of Coagulation"[4] (**Fig. 1**), which acknowledges 3 homeostatic arms. These are termed vascular, primary, and secondary hemostasis. Vascular hemostasis occurs when the vessel tissue reacts immediately to injury, such as through vasoconstriction. Primary hemostasis describes the "cellular" response and is mediated through on-site platelet activation by collagen and other factors. Secondary hemostasis includes the plasmatic contribution and describes the coagulation pathways that ultimately produce a stable fibrin lattice. Additional platelet aggregation then competes with fibrinolysis, producing a clot that ideally maximally plugs the defect while minimally occluding the lumen. Perfusion is thus restored and the stabilized vessel can begin to heal.[4] Secondary hemostasis is the only arm measured by clinical laboratory tests, and consequently laboratory data can at best only describe one piece of a complex picture.

The key mediator of secondary hemostasis is thrombin. In the cell-based theory, thrombin generation is activated initially by tissue factor (TF), which is exposed by vessel injury. TF interacts with factor VII (fVII) to form the intrinsic tenase complex, which ultimately produces a small amount of autocatalytic thrombin. Thrombin then upregulates itself in a process called the "thrombin burst," wherein thrombin performs a diverse set of hemostatic and inflammatory functions, including the activation of fV, fVIII, and fIX; the conversion of fibrinogen to soluble fibrin; direct platelet activation via the thrombin receptor; and stimulation of the immune system. Thrombin also activates anticoagulant factors to prevent runaway coagulation. A key self-regulatory step is the thrombin-activated protein C (aPC) pathway. aPC is a serine protease that (along with its cofactor protein S) targets and inhibits fVa and fVIIIa, which are key regulatory steps in the thrombin burst. Although some questions remain,[5] aPC is generally recognized as an early mediator of TIC.[6–8]

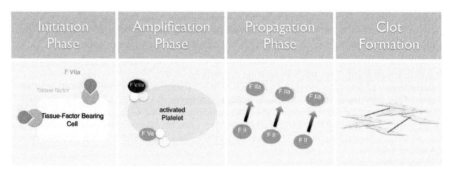

Fig. 1. The cell-based theory of coagulation. The cell-based theory of coagulation posits several phases of hemostatic activity. Initiation and amplification phases occur through interactions between platelets and the endothelium at the vessel wall. The propagation phase describes the generation of thrombin and is typically the only component of hemostasis that is measured by blood tests of coagulation.

The cell-based theory better describes in vivo hemostasis than the classic cascade model. It explains the bleeding defects observed with genetic deficiencies of factors XI, IX, and VIII, because these proteins are required for the generation of the prothrombin complex (fXa and fVa). It further defines the extrinsic and intrinsic pathways as serial, not parallel. The picture provided by this theory thereby unifies the various processes that combine to create clots that control bleeding.

TRAUMA-INDUCED COAGULOPATHY AND ACUTE TRAUMATIC COAGULOPATHY

TIC, as defined by Frith and Brohi,[2] is an umbrella term that describes the phenotype of microvascular bleeding following severe injury. The traditionally recognized components of TIC are environmental exposure (such as hypothermia), pathophysiologic processes (such as acidosis and endothelial dysfunction), and treatment complications (such as hemodilution).[2] These states are already easily diagnosed by reliable methods, such as thermometers, pH meters, and fluid balance, and do not require specific coagulation testing. The TIC syndrome also includes a newly identified hematologic pathology, called acute traumatic coagulopathy (ATC). ATC is an enzymatic process that develops rapidly after the initial traumatic impact, often before treatment has begun.[2] ATC is the specific component of TIC that is best identified and quantified by VEM.

The recognition of ATC emerged from the landmark observation by American military physicians treating combat trauma in Iraq and Afghanistan, where both higher volumes and earlier administration of plasma were associated with reduced mortality from acute hemorrhage.[9] These observations were subsequently also observed in civilian trauma,[10] although not necessarily in nontraumatic massive hemorrhage.[11,12] Although highly confounded,[13] and despite the negative results of a large multicenter trial of plasma ratios,[14] the balance of evidence has been sufficient to "move the dial," such that early factor replacement has become the standard for contemporary trauma resuscitation.[15]

The exact pathology of ATC is still under active investigation. Theusinger and colleagues[16] have shown that blood samples collected from patients at the scene of trauma (and often before further environmental exposure or any fluid resuscitation) demonstrated a marked activation of protein C, particularly with more severe trauma. Pathologic aPC was associated with reductions in fVa and fVIIIa, as expected, which characterized a specific coagulopathic process distinct from other contributors to TIC.[2] aPC may further play a role in autoheparinization,[17,18] platelet dysfunction,[19] and hyperfibrinolysis.[20] The benefits of early factor replacement might be explained by the restoration of coagulation factors opposed by aPC.

CONVENTIONAL LABORATORY ASSAYS OF COAGULATION ARE INSUFFICIENT TO DIAGNOSE ACUTE TRAUMATIC COAGULOPATHY

Perioperative hemostasis is commonly assayed by conventional laboratory testing, including the prothrombin time (PT), international normalized ratio (INR), partial thromboplastin time (PTT), fibrinogen level, and platelet count. Unfortunately, these assays have limited utility in ATC. Particularly when low diagnostic thresholds are used, the PT/INR is sensitive for ATC, but not specific,[21] and may lead to overtreatment. PTT, on the other hand, is specific but not sensitive,[22] and risks delayed diagnosis in acutely decompensating patients. Intermediate results (modestly elevated INR and normal PTT) are common and confound interpretation.[23] Quantitative fibrinogen levels and platelet counts can be determined with reasonable accuracy from conventional assays, but qualitative assays of fibrinolytic activity and platelet function are not available in most acute trauma settings.

The perfect coagulation test should be sensitive and specific. It should target many different aspects of secondary hemostasis, including both procoagulant and anticoagulant arms. It should help individualize therapy for a given patient and monitor the response to treatment. It should also be rapid, broadly interpretable, and inexpensive. That perfect laboratory test does not exist, but VEM may offer steps in that direction.

VISCOELASTIC MONITORING PLATFORMS

VEM has been used in cardiac surgery and liver transplantation for decades,[24,25] and its history and development have been elegantly reviewed elsewhere.[26] Formal use in trauma dates to a case series published in 1997.[27] Since that time, VEM platforms have become indispensable adjuncts for many trauma centers. The current version of the American College of Surgeons' Advanced Trauma Life Support recommends considering its use, although without a formal recommendation at this time.[28] Point-of-care VEM has been praised for its rapid turnaround time and personalized hemostatic profile. However, enthusiasm for these tests should not overlook their inherent limitations.

The most common VEM devices in use today are TEG and ROTEM. The best-studied TEG device is the TEG 5000 Thrombelastograph Hemostasis Analyzer (Haemonetics Corporation, Braintree, MA, USA), which is a technical update of earlier models that retains the historical rotating cup and stationary pin system. Recently, the manufacturer has introduced an ultrasound-based system called the TEG 6S (Haemonetics Corporation, Braintree, MA, USA). The technical differences between the TEG 5000 and TEG 6S have been discussed in great detail[29] and are beyond the scope of this review. Because the TEG 6S is still undergoing clinical evaluation for trauma[30] and is not yet approved for marketing for trauma by the US Food and Drug Administration (FDA) (as of 2018), this review focuses on the better studied and more widely used TEG 5000.

The best-studied ROTEM device is the ROTEM Delta (formerly TEM Innovations Gmbh, Munich, Germany, now Instrumentation Laboratory, Bedford, MA, USA). ROTEM Delta differs from the TEG 5000 primarily by rotating the pin, instead of the cup. A new cartridge-based pin system called the ROTEM Sigma (Instrumentation Laboratory, Bedford, MA, USA) is presently undergoing clinical evaluation; it does not have a 510(k) exemption by the FDA (as of 2018) and is not yet available in the United States. This discussion focuses on the ROTEM Delta platform.

Finally, other manufacturers are currently developing new hemostasis analyzers, such as the HemoSonics' Quantra (HemoSonics LLC, Charlottesville, VA, USA), but these promising devices have yet to be thoroughly investigated in trauma and will not be discussed further.

Clinicians frequently debate the merits of both TEG and ROTEM. Uncertain differences in measurements have been reported for trauma patients,[31–33] but these might be adjusted if the reference ranges were better calibrated.[32,34–36] Because meta-analyses have not demonstrated any consistent clinical differences between the TEG 5000 and ROTEM Delta,[25,37–39] including the use in trauma,[40] it is impossible to make an evidence-based statement about the superiority of either product. Under its 510(k) exemption from the UFDA, the ROTEM Delta was found to be "substantially equivalent" to the TEG 5000[41] but not superior. Therefore, we defer to the judgment of regulators that these devices are essentially identical. Some clinicians may ultimately prefer one device over another, due to marketing, technical support, theoretic benefits, institutional costs, and personal preference.[24]

THE INTERPRETATION OF VISCOELASTIC MONITORING IN TRAUMA

VEM may seem a bit challenging to interpret when seen for the first time, but users can obtain a basic literacy in a relatively short period of time. **Table 1**, **Figs. 2**, and **3** include a more complete explanation of interpretation. Separate reagents can be used to focus on specific components of clotting assays. A full description of these reagents is provided in **Table 2**.

Preclot Phase: Reaction Time and Clotting Time

The preclot phase occurs from the addition of reagents until a threshold concentration of thrombin is reached for fibrin to polymerize. With saturating agonists, this phase occurs in less than 10 minutes in a normal individual. It is measured by the reaction time (R) for TEG and the clotting time (CT) for ROTEM. If R and CT are prolonged, there may be deficiencies in clotting factors; prothrombin complex concentrates (PCCs) and plasma can be used to correct them. Because ATC affects enzymatic coagulation first, it is expected that the greatest value of VEM in trauma should be seen from prolongations of R and CT.

Factors V and VIII lie in the intrinsic pathway amplification phase, hence contact activator tests are expected to be most useful in trauma. An association between kaolin R and INTEM CT and ATC has been described,[42,43] even early into the trauma course.[44] In the laboratory, R has been shown to track with factor VIII levels.[45] In a rodent model, R was prolonged with the addition of aPC.[46] In a porcine model of dilution, prolonged R has been shown to correct with plasma transfusion,[47] suggesting that R and CT can be used to monitor the clinical response to transfusion as well.

The extrinsic pathway clotting times provide little additional information about thrombin generation beyond the intrinsic pathway tests.[42] The rapidTEG R time is generally regarded as too fast (occurring in seconds) to provide much meaningful discrimination, and so an activated clotting time (ACT) is usually substituted.[48] No studies have successfully linked the rapidTEG R with ATC. EXTEM CT has been studied in trauma and found to be inferior to the INTEM CT.[42] EXTEM CT was mildly elevated in a porcine model of untreated liver trauma,[49] which suggests some utility in that specific injury, although confirmatory studies in humans have not yet been performed. The TF assay results are available sooner (seconds vs minutes), but speed is of dubious value if the results are not useful.

Other VEM assays should not be used to evaluate thrombin generation. The FIBTEM and APTEM CT is produced by the EXTEM TF reagent, with the confounding effect of additional reagents designed to target other aspects of coagulation. The R from the TEG Functional Fibrinogen and Platelet Mapping assays are generated by exogenous reptilase and contain no information about the patient's coagulation potential.

R and CT generally do a poor job of diagnosing therapeutic anticoagulants in acute trauma patients. INR is already well studied for warfarin dosing; it is unsurprising that INR outperforms kaolin[50] and RapidTEG[51] for vitamin K antagonists. In a retrospective review of trauma patients anticoagulated with dabigatran, rivaroxaban, or apixaban, TEG performed poorly compared with calibrated anticoagulant tests and standard PT/INR and PTT.[52] VEM is not recommended as a screening test for therapeutic anticoagulation in trauma.

Clot Formation Phase: Kinetic Time, Clot Formation Time, and Alpha

Clot formation occurs from the start of fibrin polymerization until the clot reaches its maximum strength. It depends largely on fibrinogen, with some dependence on

Table 1
The major measurements derived from viscoelastic monitoring

Clotting Phase	Coagulation Step	Measurement	Interpretation in Acute Traumatic Coagulopathy	Proposed Treatment (if Clinical Coagulopathy Is Observed)
Preclot	Coagulation cascades and thrombin generation	TEG: R (reaction time) ROTEM: CT (clotting time)	If prolonged, suggests an enzymatic clotting factor deficiency	Consider clotting factor replacement with plasma or PCCs
Clot propagation	Conversion of fibrinogen to fibrin	TEG: K (kinetic time) ROTEM: CFT (clot formation time)	If prolonged, suggests an impairment in fibrinogen conversion	Consider fibrinogen replacement with plasma, cryoprecipitate, or recombinant fibrinogen
	Peak conversion of fibrinogen to fibrin	TEG and ROTEM: alpha angle	If reduced, suggests an impairment in fibrinogen conversion	
	Peak clot strength	TEG: MA (maximum amplitude) ROTEM: MCF (maximum clot firmness)	If reduced, suggests low platelet count	Consider platelet transfusion or desmopressin
Clot stability	Balance of clot formation and fibrinolysis	TEG: Ly30 (percent lysis at 30 min) ROTEM: LI (lysis index)	If increased, suggests accelerated plasmatic fibrinolysis	Consider initiation of antifibrinolytic therapy (eg, tranexamic acid)

Abbreviation: PCCs, prothrombin complex concentrates.

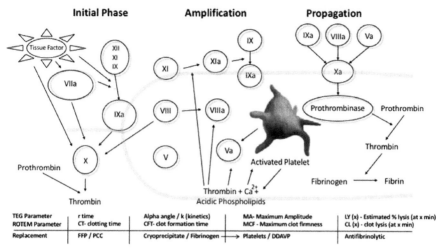

	Initial Phase	Amplification		
TEG Parameter	r time	Alpha angle / k (kinetics)	MA- Maximum Amplitude	LY (x) - Estimated % lysis (at x min)
ROTEM Parameter	CT- clotting time	CFT- clot formation time	MCF - Maximum clot firmness	CL (x) - clot lysis (at x min)
Replacement	FFP / PCC	Cryoprecipitate / Fibrinogen ⟶ Platelets / DDAVP		Antifibrinolytic

Fig. 2. Proposed physiologic events as they correlate with the viscoelastic tracing. According to VEM theory, specific points along the tracing correlate with specific phases of hemostasis, particularly the serial activation of enzymatic pathways (which ultimately generate thrombin), the formation of the early clot (largely driven by fibrin cross-linking), the full strength of the mature clot (composed of stabilized fibrin and platelets), and the early dissolution of the clot (by plasmin and other fibrinolytic mediators). (*Modified from* Pérez-Gómez F, Bover R. The new coagulation cascade and its possible influence on the delicate balance between thrombosis and hemorrhage. Rev Esp Cardiol 2007;60(12):1218. [in Spanish]; with permission.)

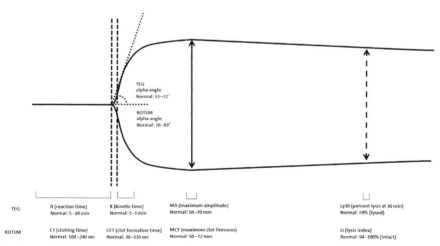

TEG	R (reaction time) Normal: 5–10 min	K (kinetic time) Normal: 1–3 min	MA (maximum amplitude) Normal: 50–70 mm	Ly30 (percent lysis at 30 min) Normal: <9% (lysed)
ROTEM	CT (clotting time) Normal: 100–240 sec	CFT (clot formation time) Normal: 30–110 sec	MCF (maximum clot firmness) Normal: 50–72 mm	LI (lysis index) Normal: 94–100% (intact)

Fig. 3. Interpreting the generic viscoelastic tracing. The generic VEM tracing serves as the basis for the individual measurements provided by the VEM platforms. The R and CT are measured from the start of the assay until the lines diverge by 2 mm, and the C and CFT are measured when the divergence reaches 20 mm. The alpha angle is derived from the angle of incidence formed by a line connecting the origin of the line divergence and the inflection point of the tracing curves. The MA and MCF are measured by the widest divergence of the lines. The Ly30 and LI are measured by the percentage of narrowing of the lines over a 30 minute interval.

Table 2
Specific types of VEM assays and reagents

Assay Target	TEG	ROTEM	Comments
"Native"	No reagents	No reagents	High variability, generally not used clinically
Intrinsic activation	Kaolin TEG	INTEM (ellagic acid)	R and CT reflect the "thrombin burst"
Extrinsic activation	RapidTEG (tissue factor)	EXTEM (tissue factor)	R and CT reflect factor VII activity primarily; all other VEM parameters generally identical to intrinsic pathway but are provided sooner
Fibrinogen level	TEG Functional Fibrinogen (reptilase and abciximab)	FIBTEM (EXTEM and cytochalasin D)	Potent antiplatelet reagents ensure that the MA and MCF primarily reflect fibrin contribution; may provide better measurement of fibrinogen level than standard K, CFT, and alpha
Platelet function	TEG Platelet Mapping (heparin, reptilase, rFXIII, either ADP or arachidonic acid)	None (ROTEM platelet is an aggregometric assay)	Returns a percent inhibition of the ADP and thromboxane A_2 pathways; intended by manufacturer to facilitate dosing dual antiplatelet therapy (specifically clopidogrel and aspirin); not validated as a diagnostic test of platelet function
Fibrinolysis/antifibrinolytic effect	None	APTEM (EXTEM and aprotinin)	Correction of LI by aprotinin thought to indicate the presence of hyperfibrinolysis with greater sensitivity than standard LI
Residual heparin	Heparinase TEG (heparin, kaolin)	HEPTEM (INTEM and protamine)	Correction of R and CT by heparin antagonists thought to indicate residual heparin anticoagulation; generally not used for trauma

Abbreviation: ADP, adenosine diphosphate.

thrombin, functional platelets, and factor XIII. This phase is measured by K (kinetic time) for TEG, CFT (clot formation time) for ROTEM, and alpha angle for both devices. Prolongation of K and CFT, or reduction in alpha, suggest a fibrinogen deficiency that can be treated with cryoprecipitate or fibrinogen concentrates.

VEM has generally not been shown to alter fibrinogen replacement in trauma. In meta-analyses, K, CFT, and alpha do not change rates of cryoprecipitate use, bleeding, or mortality.[25,37,38] K, CFT, and alpha are all susceptible to confounding in the setting of reduced thrombin generation[49,53] and low platelets[54] and can be difficult to interpret in complex bleeding states.[55] For trauma, these studies are complicated by small sample size, study site variation, and bias.[40] Absent any theoretic or clinical correlation with ATC, treatment decisions based on these VEM numbers should be made carefully, with the further recognition that plasma transfusions also replace fibrinogen, although not as effectively as concentrates.[56]

K, CFT, and alpha values obtained from the TF assays (rapidTEG and EXTEM) seem to correlate well with contact activator VEMs (kaolin TEG and INTEM).[57] As expected, results can be obtained faster, saving approximately 5 to 6 minutes,[58] although the time difference may not be clinically significant.

The diagnostic accuracy of VEM for fibrinogen deficiencies might be improved by the addition of fibrin-specific assays, such as the TEG Functional Fibrinogen and the ROTEM FIBTEM. At least one in vitro study found that Functional Fibrinogen could predict hypofibrinogenemia (in plasma supplemented with fibrinogen concentrate) better than the standard alpha angle alone.[54] The Functional Fibrinogen MA and FIB-TEM MCF have been shown to track with the fibrinogen level more closely than the standard K, CFT, and alpha[55] and may also predict mortality[55,59] but have not been shown to improve clinical outcomes. It should be remembered that the laboratory-based fibrinogen remains the gold standard measurement to which VEM is compared, and fibrinogen levels are preferred whenever available.

Clot Strength: Maximum Amplitude and Maximum Clot Firmness

Total clot strength is measured by the maximum amplitude (MA) for TEG and maximum clot firmness (MCF) for ROTEM, and it has been associated with platelet count (although up to 20% of the MA and MCF is due to fibrin). Low MA and MCF are often treated with platelet transfusions. Clot stabilization occurs after the MA and MCF are reached, when enzymatic fibrinolysis may declare itself.

Reductions in MA and MCF can be seen early in major trauma and may predict worse outcomes.[55,60] TF and contact activator agonists produce similar MA and MCF measurements.[42] As for the K and CFT, rapidTEG and EXTEM return the MA and MCF approximately 6 minutes faster (on average) than kaolin TEG and INTEM,[58,61] although this difference can be mitigated if clinicians interpret the A5 and A10 measurements.[62] The measurements depend to some degree on fibrin polymerization and thrombin generation,[24,26] and so they are modestly confounded by defects in other pathways.

In trauma, MA- and MCF-guided platelet algorithms have been shown to increase the volume[63] and reduce the time to platelet transfusion.[62,64] Increased utilization stands in stark contrast to the generally platelet-saving effect of VEM in cardiac surgery and liver transplantation.[25,37,38] A possible explanation may be a bias for empirical plasma over empirical platelets at some institutions, in which case a rapid MA or MCF result can trigger early transfusion.

MA and MCF are only correlated with the platelet count.[63] As with fibrinogen, clinicians should defer to the gold-standard platelet count whenever it is available, provided that the results can be returned in a clinically meaningful time. MA and MCF may have value as a quick estimate of platelet count when an answer (even an imprecise one) is required urgently.

There is emerging interest in the use of TEG Platelet Mapping in trauma. The commercial kit includes reagents for the adenosine diphosphate and (the thromboxane A_2-precursor) arachidonic acid pathways. The ROTEM platelet test also measures these pathways but (despite the ROTEM branding) is an aggregometric technique and is not a VEM method. These pathways were selected to assist dosing clopidogrel and aspirin for dual antiplatelet therapy and are not intended for disease diagnosis. Indeed, the variability in the healthy population is so great that a reference range has yet to be established.[65] The arachidonic acid agonist in the Platelet Mapping kit may have some utility to rule-out COX-1 inhibitors in traumatic brain injury,[66] but more investigation should be performed before these results should trigger treatment decisions. Retrospective analysis has failed to find an association between Platelet Mapping and ATC.[67,68] The use of Platelet Mapping is speculative at best and may lead to overtreatment due to a high false-positive rate.

Fibrinolysis: Ly30 and LI

VEM stands out as the only diagnostic tool available to most perioperative physicians for the detection of hyperfibrinolysis. Overall, hyperfibrinolysis is relatively rare in trauma,[69] but its consequences are dire, including a several-fold increased risk of death.[40,70–73] Fibrinolysis can be managed effectively with inexpensive, relatively safe, antifibrinolytic medications, such as tranexamic acid.

Fibrinolysis is measured by the Ly30 and LI, both of which measure the degree of clot narrowing that occurs over 30 minutes. In meta-analyses, Ly30 and LI have not been shown to improve any clinical outcome or increase the use of antifibrinolytic agents,[25,37,38,40] but sample sizes include too few patients with hyperfibrinolysis for sufficient power. Although false-positive cases are unlikely to experience harm from overtreatment, the consequences of undertreatment of false negatives could be disastrous. Therefore, absent better data, it would be prudent to treat hyperfibrinolysis aggressively whenever detected by VEM or when microvascular bleeding persists despite a normal Ly30 or LI.

Low Ly30 and LI (eg, <3%) have been argued to predict "fibrinolytic shutdown," wherein fibrinolysis is reduced (rather than activated) in ATC.[74] Interpretation of those results is unclear, with discordant findings.[74,75] Until more data are available, a "low" Ly30 or LI should not trigger treatment.

The APTEM assay is a specialized ROTEM assay for fibrinolysis. APTEM has not yet been studied in the setting of ATC, and its value is unknown.

VISCOELASTIC MONITORING PROTOCOLS AND CLINICAL OUTCOMES
Blood Products

The greatest benefit seen from VEM across all indications is seen when it is used to inform plasma and PCC use. In meta-analyses of VEM across all indications (although largely driven by cardiac surgery), the most consistent and prominent reductions in blood product use (perhaps as much as 50%) are seen for plasma transfusions.[25,37,38]

In retrospective studies and clinical trials, VEM is generally treated as a blood-saving technology. Literature most strongly suggests that VEM protocols reduce transfusions.[76–78] The greatest benefit is typically seen for reductions in the plasma level and PCCs, by perhaps as much as 50%.[78,79] Although some investigators have reported increased blood product consumption after instituting VEM,[80] their findings cannot be separated from local interpretations of strict VEM protocols and probably represent overtreatment.[81] At centers where the alternative to VEM in trauma is the empirical use of 1:1 transfusion ratios, some of which will be administered to patients without ATC, then the added ability that VEM adds to distinguish patients who would benefit from plasma from who would not.[76,82,83] VEM should be expected to reduce overtreatment. Its value to prevent undertreatment is expected only for centers with more conservative transfusion practices that tend to underdiagnose ATC. Therefore, the results from studies showing evolutions in local transfusion practice after installing VEM highly depend on the local practice and may not be replicable where practices differ.

Mortality

One limitation of VEM is the consistent failure to demonstrate reductions in mortality. Most meta-analyses have failed to find any mortality benefit across all indications.[37–40] Although one recent meta-analysis suggested improved survival, it was seen only when including studies that used a traditional laboratory or placebo controls; the same meta-analysis was unable to demonstrate improved mortality over "usual care," which includes clinician judgment and empirical plasma:RBC ratio massive transfusions.[25] Only one prospective trial (Gonzalez and colleagues[84]) reported modestly improved survival ($P = .049$) using a rapidTEG protocol, which provided a massive transfusion protocol for an abnormal ACT rather than VEM specifically. The control group was not transfused until conventional laboratory data were available, which can be delayed by 30 minutes at the study site,[85] and delayed treatment is independently associated with mortality.[86] Based on these studies, it would seem that unconstrained clinicians save lives just as well without VEM.[24]

Providers may question whether it is important for studies to demonstrate a mortality benefit at all. The benefit of VEM (or any laboratory test) is not mortality but the correct identification of which patients will benefit from transfusion and which will not.[24] Results suggesting cost-effectiveness,[38] reduced transfusions,[25,38] and shorter length-of-stay[87] should be sufficient to justify the use of VEM in trauma. Mortality may not be necessary at all for clinicians to adopt VEM into their practice, if the ancillary benefits are strong.

SUMMARY

TEG and ROTEM are imperfect assays, but they are certainly not useless. They provide additional diagnostic information in confusing and chaotic environments. Clinicians should focus on those numbers that provide the greatest diagnostic discrimination. For TEG, this includes R from kaolin, MA, and Ly30. For ROTEM, this includes the CT from INTEM, MCF, and LI. Functional Fibrinogen and FIBTEM may also be useful, after more investigation. VEM is preferable to PT/INR and PTT, but clinicians should defer to fibrinogen and platelet counts when they are available. VEM may not improve mortality but may accelerate targeted hemostatic resuscitation. Lastly, one needs to consider the near-impossibility of designing and executing a meaningful prospective trial for interventions (and especially a laboratory test) in the heterogenous trauma population. We may never have solid and definitive data to support the use of VEM in trauma and may have to accept lower quality evidence about its use.

REFERENCES

1. Brohi K, Singh J, Heron M, et al. Acute traumatic coagulopathy. J Trauma 2003; 54(6):1127–30.
2. Frith D, Davenport R, Brohi K. Acute traumatic coagulopathy. Curr Opin Anaesthesiol 2012;25(2):229–34.

3. Harris T, Davenport R, Mak M, et al. The evolving science of trauma resuscitation. Emerg Med Clin North Am 2018;36(1):85–106.
4. Hoffman M, Monroe DM 3rd. A cell-based model of hemostasis. Thromb Haemost 2001;85(6):958–65.
5. Gando S, Mayumi T, Ukai T. Activated protein C plays no major roles in the inhibition of coagulation or increased fibrinolysis in acute coagulopathy of trauma-shock: a systematic review. Thromb J 2018;16:13.
6. Cohen MJ, Call M, Nelson M, et al. Critical role of activated protein C in early coagulopathy and later organ failure, infection and death in trauma patients. Ann Surg 2012;255(2):379–85.
7. Davenport RA, Guerreiro M, Frith D, et al. Activated protein C drives the hyperfibrinolysis of acute traumatic coagulopathy. Anesthesiology 2017;126(1):115–27.
8. Davenport RA, Brohi K. Cause of trauma-induced coagulopathy. Curr Opin Anaesthesiol 2016;29(2):212–9.
9. Borgman MA, Spinella PC, Perkins JG, et al. The ratio of blood products transfused affects mortality in patients receiving massive transfusions at a combat support hospital. J Trauma 2007;63(4):805–13.
10. Holcomb JB, Wade CE, Michalek JE, et al. Increased plasma and platelet to red blood cell ratios improves outcome in 466 massively transfused civilian trauma patients. Ann Surg 2008;248(3):447–58.
11. Inaba K, Branco BC, Rhee P, et al. Impact of plasma transfusion in trauma patients who do not require massive transfusion. J Am Coll Surg 2010;210(6): 957–65.
12. McQuilten ZK, Crighton G, Brunskill S, et al. Optimal dose, timing and ratio of blood products in massive transfusion: results from a systematic review. Transfus Med Rev 2018;32(1):6–15.
13. Ho AM, Dion PW, Yeung JH, et al. Prevalence of survivor bias in observational studies on fresh frozen plasma:erythrocyte ratios in trauma requiring massive transfusion. Anesthesiology 2012;116(3):716–28.
14. Holcomb JB, Tilley BC, Baraniuk S, et al. Transfusion of plasma, platelets, and red blood cells in a 1:1:1 vs a 1:1:2 ratio and mortality in patients with severe trauma: the PROPPR randomized clinical trial. JAMA 2015;313(5):471–82.
15. Hess JR, Ramos PJ, Sen NE, et al. Quality management of a massive transfusion protocol. Transfusion 2018;58(2):480–4.
16. Theusinger OM, Baulig W, Seifert B, et al. Changes in coagulation in standard laboratory tests and ROTEM in trauma patients between on-scene and arrival in the emergency department. Anesth Analg 2015;120(3):627–35.
17. Ostrowski SR, Johansson PI. Endothelial glycocalyx degradation induces endogenous heparinization in patients with severe injury and early traumatic coagulopathy. J Trauma Acute Care Surg 2012;73(1):60–6.
18. Kettner SC, Gonano C, Seebach F, et al. Endogenous heparin-like substances significantly impair coagulation in patients undergoing orthotopic liver transplantation. Anesth Analg 1998;86(4):691–5.
19. Stavenuiter F, Davis NF, Duan E, et al. Platelet protein S directly inhibits procoagulant activity on platelets and microparticles. Thromb Haemost 2013;109(2): 229–37.
20. Theusinger OM, Wanner GA, Emmert MY, et al. Hyperfibrinolysis diagnosed by rotational thromboelastometry (ROTEM) is associated with higher mortality in patients with severe trauma. Anesth Analg 2011;113(5):1003–12.

21. McCully SP, Fabricant LJ, Kunio NR, et al. The International Normalized Ratio overestimates coagulopathy in stable trauma and surgical patients. J Trauma Acute Care Surg 2013;75(6):947–53.

22. Rugeri L, Levrat A, David JS, et al. Diagnosis of early coagulation abnormalities in trauma patients by rotation thrombelastography. J Thromb Haemost 2007;5(2): 289–95.

23. MacLeod JB, Lynn M, McKenney MG, et al. Early coagulopathy predicts mortality in trauma. J Trauma 2003;55(1):39–44.

24. Blaine KP, Sakai T. Viscoelastic monitoring to guide hemostatic resuscitation in liver transplantation surgery. Semin Cardiothorac Vasc Anesth 2018;22(2): 150–63.

25. Wikkelso A, Wetterslev J, Moller AM, et al. Thromboelastography (TEG) or thromboelastometry (ROTEM) to monitor haemostatic treatment versus usual care in adults or children with bleeding. Cochrane Database Syst Rev 2016;(8):CD007871.

26. Hochleitner G, Sutor K, Levett C, et al. Revisiting Hartert's 1962 calculation of the physical constants of thrombelastography. Clin Appl Thromb Hemost 2017;23(3): 201–10.

27. Kaufmann CR, Dwyer KM, Crews JD, et al. Usefulness of thrombelastography in assessment of trauma patient coagulation. J Trauma 1997;42(4):716–20 [discussion: 720–2].

28. American College of Surgeons Committee on Trauma. Advanced trauma life support: student course manual. 10th edition. Chicago (IL): American College of Surgeons; 2018.

29. Gurbel PA, Bliden KP, Tantry US, et al. First report of the point-of-care TEG: a technical validation study of the TEG-6S system. Platelets 2016;27(7):642–9.

30. Meledeo MA, Peltier GC, McIntosh CS, et al. Functional stability of the TEG 6s hemostasis analyzer under stress. J Trauma Acute Care Surg 2018;84(6S Suppl 1): S83–8.

31. Hagemo JS, Naess PA, Johansson P, et al. Evaluation of TEG((R)) and Ro-TEM((R)) inter-changeability in trauma patients. Injury 2013;44(5):600–5.

32. Sankarankutty A, Nascimento B, Teodoro da Luz L, et al. TEG(R) and ROTEM(R) in trauma: similar test but different results? World J Emerg Surg 2012;7(Suppl 1):S3.

33. Rizoli S, Min A, Sanchez AP, et al. In trauma, conventional ROTEM and TEG results are not interchangeable but are similar in clinical applicability. Mil Med 2016;181(5 Suppl):117–26.

34. Scarpelini S, Rhind SG, Nascimento B, et al. Normal range values for thromboelastography in healthy adult volunteers. Braz J Med Biol Res 2009;42(12):1210–7.

35. Lier H, Vorweg M, Hanke A, et al. Thromboelastometry guided therapy of severe bleeding. Essener Runde algorithm. Hamostaseologie 2013;33(1):51–61.

36. Baksaas-Aasen K, Van Dieren S, Balvers K, et al. Data-driven development of ROTEM and TEG algorithms for the management of trauma hemorrhage: a prospective observational multicenter study. Ann Surg 2018. [Epub ahead of print].

37. Corredor C, Thomson R, Al-Subaie N. Long-term consequences of acute kidney injury after cardiac surgery: a systematic review and meta-analysis J Cardiothorac Vasc Anesth 2016;30(1):69–75.

38. Whiting P, Al M, Westwood M, et al. Viscoelastic point-of-care testing to assist with the diagnosis, management and monitoring of haemostasis: a systematic review and cost-effectiveness analysis. Health Technol Assess 2015;19(58):1–228, v-vi.

39. Fahrendorff M, Oliveri RS, Johansson PI. The use of viscoelastic haemostatic assays in goal-directing treatment with allogeneic blood products - A systematic review and meta-analysis. Scand J Trauma Resusc Emerg Med 2017;25(1):39.
40. Hunt H, Stanworth S, Curry N, et al. Thromboelastography (TEG) and rotational thromboelastometry (ROTEM) for trauma induced coagulopathy in adult trauma patients with bleeding. Cochrane Database Syst Rev 2015;(2):CD010438.
41. US Food and Drug Administration. 510(k) substantial equivalence determination decision summary. Center for Devices and Radiological Health. 2010. Available at: https://www.accessdata.fda.gov/scripts/cdrh/cfdocs/cfpmn/pmn.cfm?ID=K101533.
42. Harr JN, Moore EE, Chin TL, et al. Viscoelastic hemostatic fibrinogen assays detect fibrinolysis early. Eur J Trauma Emerg Surg 2015;41(1):49–56.
43. Kane I, Ong A, Orozco FR, et al. Thromboelastography predictive of death in trauma patients. Orthop Surg 2015;7(1):26–30.
44. Duan K, Yu W, Lin Z, et al. A time course study of acute traumatic coagulopathy prior to resuscitation: from hypercoagulation to hypocoagulation caused by hypoperfusion? Transfus Apher Sci 2014;50(3):399–406.
45. Golder M, Mewburn J, Lillicrap D. In vitro and in vivo evaluation of the effect of elevated factor VIII on the thrombogenic process. Thromb Haemost 2013; 109(1):53–60.
46. Harr JN, Moore EE, Wohlauer MV, et al. The acute coagulopathy of trauma is due to impaired initial thrombin generation but not clot formation or clot strength. J Surg Res 2011;170(2):319–24.
47. Kostousov V, Wang YW, Wade CE, et al. Hemostatically distinct FFPs equally improve abnormal TEG variables in an in vitro dilutional coagulopathy model. Thromb Res 2012;130(3):429–34.
48. Moore HB, Moore EE, Chin TL, et al. Activated clotting time of thrombelastography (T-ACT) predicts early postinjury blood component transfusion beyond plasma. Surgery 2014;156(3):564–9.
49. Zentai C, Solomon C, van der Meijden PE, et al. Effects of fibrinogen concentrate on thrombin generation, thromboelastometry parameters, and laboratory coagulation testing in a 24-hour porcine trauma model. Clin Appl Thromb Hemost 2016; 22(8):749–59.
50. Nascimento B, Al Mahoos M, Callum J, et al. Vitamin K-dependent coagulation factor deficiency in trauma: a comparative analysis between international normalized ratio and thromboelastography. Transfusion 2012;52(1):7–13.
51. Dunham CM, Rabel C, Hileman BM, et al. TEG(R) and RapidTEG(R) are unreliable for detecting warfarin-coagulopathy: a prospective cohort study. Thromb J 2014;12(1):4.
52. Ali JT, Daley MJ, Vadiei N, et al. Thromboelastogram does not detect pre-injury anticoagulation in acute trauma patients. Am J Emerg Med 2017;35(4):632–6.
53. Jeger V, Willi S, Liu T, et al. The rapid TEG alpha-angle may be a sensitive predictor of transfusion in moderately injured blunt trauma patients. ScientificWorldJournal 2012;2012:821794.
54. Solomon C, Schochl H, Ranucci M, et al. Can the viscoelastic parameter alpha-angle distinguish fibrinogen from platelet deficiency and guide fibrinogen supplementation? Anesth Analg 2015;121(2):289–301.
55. Harr JN, Moore EE, Ghasabyan A, et al. Functional fibrinogen assay indicates that fibrinogen is critical in correcting abnormal clot strength following trauma. Shock 2013;39(1):45–9.
56. Franchini M, Lippi G. Fibrinogen replacement therapy: a critical review of the literature. Blood Transfus 2012;10(1):23–7.

57. Da Luz LT, Nascimento B, Shankarakutty AK, et al. Effect of thromboelastography (TEG(R)) and rotational thromboelastometry (ROTEM(R)) on diagnosis of coagulopathy, transfusion guidance and mortality in trauma: descriptive systematic review. Crit Care 2014;18(5):518.

58. Cotton BA, Faz G, Hatch QM, et al. Rapid thrombelastography delivers real-time results that predict transfusion within 1 hour of admission. J Trauma 2011;71(2): 407–14 [discussion: 414–7].

59. Tauber H, Innerhofer P, Breitkopf R, et al. Prevalence and impact of abnormal ROTEM(R) assays in severe blunt trauma: results of the 'diagnosis and treatment of trauma-induced coagulopathy (DIA-TRE-TIC) study'. Br J Anaesth 2011;107(3): 378–87.

60. Nystrup KB, Windelov NA, Thomsen AB, et al. Reduced clot strength upon admission, evaluated by thrombelastography (TEG), in trauma patients is independently associated with increased 30-day mortality. Scand J Trauma Resusc Emerg Med 2011;19:52.

61. Meyer AS, Meyer MA, Sorensen AM, et al. Thrombelastography and rotational thromboelastometry early amplitudes in 182 trauma patients with clinical suspicion of severe injury. J Trauma Acute Care Surg 2014;76(3):682–90.

62. Laursen TH, Meyer MAS, Meyer ASP, et al. Thrombelastography early amplitudes in bleeding and coagulopathic trauma patients: results from a multicenter study. J Trauma Acute Care Surg 2018;84(2):334–41.

63. Plotkin AJ, Wade CE, Jenkins DH, et al. A reduction in clot formation rate and strength assessed by thrombelastography is indicative of transfusion requirements in patients with penetrating injuries. J Trauma 2008;64(2 Suppl):S64–8.

64. Johansson PI, Sorensen AM, Larsen CF, et al. Low hemorrhage-related mortality in trauma patients in a Level I trauma center employing transfusion packages and early thromboelastography-directed hemostatic resuscitation with plasma and platelets. Transfusion 2013;53(12):3088–99.

65. Bochsen L, Wiinberg B, Kjelgaard-Hansen M, et al. Evaluation of the TEG platelet mapping assay in blood donors. Thromb J 2007;5:3.

66. Connelly CR, Yonge JD, McCully SP, et al. Assessment of three point-of-care platelet function assays in adult trauma patients. J Surg Res 2017;212:260–9.

67. George MJ, Burchfield J, MacFarlane B, et al. Multiplate and TEG platelet mapping in a population of severely injured trauma patients. Transfus Med 2018; 28(3):224–30.

68. Daley MJ, Trust MD, Peterson EJ, et al. Thromboelastography does not detect preinjury antiplatelet therapy in acute trauma patients. Am Surg 2016;82(2): 175–80.

69. Ostrowski SR, Sorensen AM, Larsen CF, et al. Thrombelastography and biomarker profiles in acute coagulopathy of trauma: a prospective study. Scand J Trauma Resusc Emerg Med 2011;19:64.

70. Chapman MP, Moore EE, Moore HB, et al. The "Death Diamond": rapid thrombelastography identifies lethal hyperfibrinolysis. J Trauma Acute Care Surg 2015; 79(6):925–9.

71. Cotton BA, Harvin JA, Kostousouv V, et al. Hyperfibrinolysis at admission is an uncommon but highly lethal event associated with shock and prehospital fluid administration. J Trauma Acute Care Surg 2012;73(2):365–70 [discussion: 370].

72. Taylor JR 3rd, Fox EE, Holcomb JB, et al. The hyperfibrinolytic phenotype is the most lethal and resource intense presentation of fibrinolysis in massive transfusion patients. J Trauma Acute Care Surg 2018;84(1):25–30.

73. Schochl H, Frietsch T, Pavelka M, et al. Hyperfibrinolysis after major trauma: differential diagnosis of lysis patterns and prognostic value of thrombelastometry. J Trauma 2009;67(1):125–31.
74. Gomez-Builes JC, Acuna SA, Nascimento B, et al. Harmful or physiologic: diagnosing fibrinolysis shutdown in a trauma cohort with rotational thromboelastometry. Anesth Analg 2018;127(4):840–9.
75. Kashuk JL, Moore EE, Sawyer M, et al. Primary fibrinolysis is integral in the pathogenesis of the acute coagulopathy of trauma. Ann Surg 2010;252(3):434–42 [discussion: 443–4].
76. Yin J, Zhao Z, Li Y, et al. Goal-directed transfusion protocol via thrombelastography in patients with abdominal trauma: a retrospective study. World J Emerg Surg 2014;9:28.
77. Schochl H, Nienaber U, Maegele M, et al. Transfusion in trauma: thromboelastometry-guided coagulation factor concentrate-based therapy versus standard fresh frozen plasma-based therapy. Crit Care 2011;15(2):R83.
78. Gorlinger K, Fries D, Dirkmann D, et al. Reduction of fresh frozen plasma requirements by perioperative point-of-care coagulation management with early calculated goal-directed therapy. Transfus Med Hemother 2012;39(2):104–13.
79. Nienaber U, Innerhofer P, Westermann I, et al. The impact of fresh frozen plasma vs coagulation factor concentrates on morbidity and mortality in trauma-associated haemorrhage and massive transfusion. Injury 2011;42(7):697–701.
80. Holcomb JB, Minei KM, Scerbo ML, et al. Admission rapid thrombelastography can replace conventional coagulation tests in the emergency department: experience with 1974 consecutive trauma patients. Ann Surg 2012;256(3):476–86.
81. Chang R, Fox EE, Greene TJ, et al. Abnormalities of laboratory coagulation tests versus clinically evident coagulopathic bleeding: results from the prehospital resuscitation on helicopters study (PROHS). Surgery 2018;163(4):819–26.
82. Tapia NM, Chang A, Norman M, et al. TEG-guided resuscitation is superior to standardized MTP resuscitation in massively transfused penetrating trauma patients. J Trauma Acute Care Surg 2013;74(2):378–85 [discussion: 385–6].
83. Howley IW, Haut ER, Jacobs L, et al. Is thromboelastography (TEG)-based resuscitation better than empirical 1:1 transfusion? Trauma Surg Acute Care Open 2018;3(1):e000140.
84. Gonzalez E, Moore EE, Moore HB, et al. Goal-directed hemostatic resuscitation of trauma-induced coagulopathy: a pragmatic randomized clinical trial comparing a viscoelastic assay to conventional coagulation assays. Ann Surg 2016;263(6):1051–9.
85. Pezold M, Moore EE, Wohlauer M, et al. Viscoelastic clot strength predicts coagulation-related mortality within 15 minutes. Surgery 2012;151(1):48–54.
86. Spahn DR. TEG(R)- or ROTEM(R)-based individualized goal-directed coagulation algorithms: don't wait–act now! Crit Care 2014;18(6):637.
87. Wang H, Robinson RD, Phillips JL, et al. Traumatic abdominal solid organ injury patients might benefit from thromboelastography-guided blood component therapy. J Clin Med Res 2017;9(5):433–8.

Enhanced Recovery After Surgery

Are the Principles Applicable to Adult and Geriatric Acute Care and Trauma Surgery?

Mandeep Singh, MD[a],*, Reza Askari, MD[b],
Matthias Stopfkuchen-Evans, MD[c]

KEYWORDS

- Enhanced recovery • Elderly • Urgent surgery • Perioperative care

KEY POINTS

- The enhanced recovery after surgery (ERAS®) guidelines were formulated in 2012 in colonic, pelvic or rectal, and pancreatic surgery with a goal of decreasing hospital length of stay and time to resumption of normal activities while improving survival with preoperative, intraoperative, and postoperative management recommendations.
- Most geriatric patients undergoing ERAS-based perioperative care show no differences in comparison with younger adults in terms of postoperative time to passage of flatus, advancement of diet, removal of Foley catheter, complications, and length of postoperative stay, while also experiencing less delirium compared with non-ERAS care.
- Incorporating ERAS principles in the adult or geriatric acute care surgery patient populations has been shown in multiple research studies to minimize time to resumption of preoperative activity in addition to reducing hospital length of stay.
- ERAS principles are widely applicable to adult or geriatric acute care surgery patient populations, whereas in trauma patients the current evidence base is limited. Increased physician and nursing education to use enhanced recovery protocols will further improve quality of health care administered in the twenty-first century.

Disclosures: None.
Funding Sources: None.
Conflicts of Interest: None.
[a] Cardiothoracic Anesthesiology and Critical Care, Department of Anesthesiology, Keck Medical Center, University of Southern California, 1450 San Pablo Street, Suite 3600, Los Angeles, CA 90033, USA; [b] Department of Surgery, Brigham and Women's Hospital, Harvard Medical School, 75 Francis Street, Boston, MA 02115, USA; [c] Department of Anesthesiology, Brigham and Women's Hospital, Harvard Medical School, 75 Francis Street, CWN L1, Boston, MA 02115, USA
* Corresponding author.
E-mail address: Mandeep.singh@med.usc.edu

INTRODUCTION

Enhanced recovery after surgery (ERAS) principles comprise various perioperative protocols that have been developed to reduce recovery time and promote a patient's return to normal or preoperative function. The ERAS philosophy aims to increase physiologic reserve, reduce perioperative stress, and restore organ function rapidly after surgery through these protocols. Although the implementation of the protocols' key preoperative and postoperative principles is less challenging with scheduled, elective surgical procedures, many perioperative protocol components may also be incorporated in adult or geriatric acute care and trauma surgery to improve surgical outcomes. This review discusses evidence-based recommendations and the key ERAS principles that can be implemented in the adult or geriatric acute care surgery setting and probably in trauma surgery.

BACKGROUND

Emergency and trauma surgeries often result in complications and extended hospital stays for adult or geriatric patients.[1] The ERAS movement is inspired by the work of the notable Danish surgeon Henrik Kehlet, who questioned the benefit of standard care measures for surgical patients, such as mechanical bowel preparation, gradual resumption of diet, extended preoperative fasting, and delayed ambulation. Kehlet postulated that the avoidance of such measures would actually reduce metabolic stress on the patient and shorten hospital length of stay.[2] An ERAS® protocol of 20 items was ultimately created by an international ERAS study group (including both surgeons and anesthesiologists) to optimize perioperative care of the surgical patient. In 2012, the ERAS® Society, the European Society of Clinical Nutrition and Metabolism, and the International Association for Surgical Metabolism and Nutrition, issued updated consensus recommendations: ERAS in colonic,[3] pelvic or rectal,[4] and pancreatic surgery,[5] with a goal of decreasing hospital length of stay and time to resumption of normal activities while improving survival.[6,7] ERAS has been shown to reduce surgical complication rates and be a cost-effective methodology for reducing health care and hospital costs.[8,9]

The ERAS care plan is divided into preoperative, intraoperative, and postoperative management recommendations (**Fig. 1**).[2]

Preoperative considerations include preadmission education, early discharge planning, selective choice of patients receiving bowel preparation, antibiotic prophylaxis, prewarming, deep venous thrombosis prophylaxis, carbohydrate loading, and reduced fasting duration. Preadmission education aims to reduce patient stress and anxiety related to the surgery, and motivates the patient to adhere to postoperative pain and physical therapy management protocols.[5] Prolonged starvation greater than 8 hours for solids and 2 hours for carbohydrate-containing liquids has been shown to place patients in a catabolic metabolic state, which has been associated with prolonged hospital stay and increased insulin resistance that is worsened by perioperative cortisol and stress hormone release.[6] Increased insulin resistance reduces muscle glucose intake and contributes to reduced muscle mass and strength, which is particularly important in the postoperative recovery setting; hyperglycemia also increases the risk of infection. Preoperative carbohydrate loading has been correlated with reduced insulin resistance and has not been associated with increased aspiration risk.[10,11] Patients undergoing major abdominal surgery with these guidelines have had reductions in hospital stay by 1 day.[12] Bowel preparation has widely been abandoned because it causes electrolyte imbalances, such as hypocalcemia and hypophosphatemia, in addition to anastomotic leakage.[13,14]

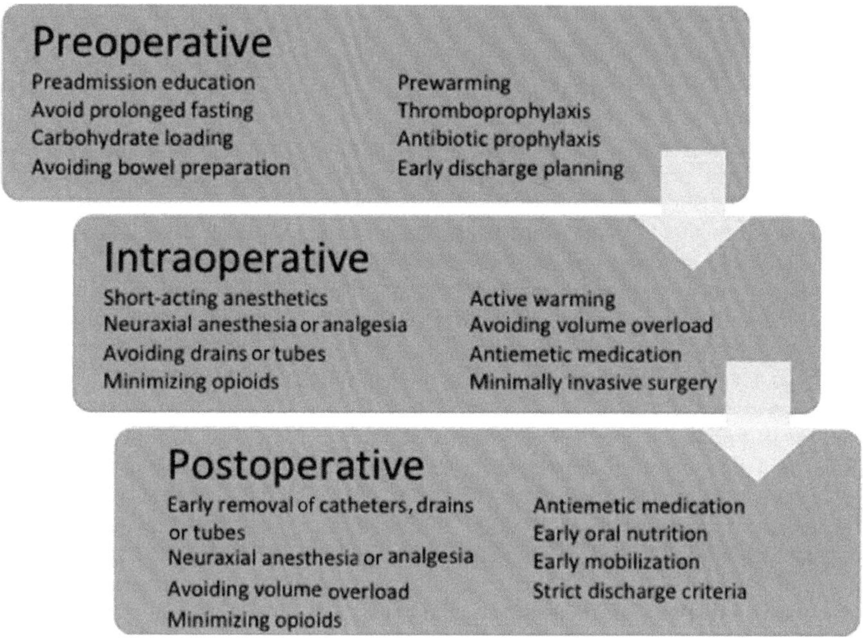

Preoperative

Preadmission education
Avoid prolonged fasting
Carbohydrate loading
Avoiding bowel preparation

Prewarming
Thromboprophylaxis
Antibiotic prophylaxis
Early discharge planning

Intraoperative

Short-acting anesthetics
Neuraxial anesthesia or analgesia
Avoiding drains or tubes
Minimizing opioids

Active warming
Avoiding volume overload
Antiemetic medication
Minimally invasive surgery

Postoperative

Early removal of catheters, drains
or tubes
Neuraxial anesthesia or analgesia
Avoiding volume overload
Minimizing opioids

Antiemetic medication
Early oral nutrition
Early mobilization
Strict discharge criteria

Fig. 1. Typical ERAS® protocol (eg, elective colorectal surgery).

Intraoperative considerations include active warming techniques (eg, forced air warming, use of warmed intravenous fluids), using minimally invasive rather than open surgical techniques, minimizing opioid use, avoiding prophylactic nasogastric tubes and drains (which are associated with fever, impaired mobility, pneumonia), incorporating pain and nausea prophylaxis, and using goal-directed fluid management. Maintaining normal body temperature reduces bleeding and transfusion requirements, along with reducing infection rates and incidence of cardiac arrhythmias.[15] Older intravenous fluid administration regimens incorporated large volumes that often exceeded actual or measured fluid losses,[16] with patients sometimes receiving up to 7 L of fluids intraoperatively for routine abdominal surgery and up to 3 L postoperatively.[17,18] Such liberal administration of intravenous fluids results in damage to the endothelial glycocalyx and accumulation of fluid in the interstitial space with complications such as delayed wound healing and prolonged return of normal bowel function. Administering large volumes of normal saline may case hyperchloremic acidosis and increase the risk of acute kidney injury. Individuals with risk factors for postoperative nausea and vomiting (eg, young female patients, nonsmokers) should receive antiemetic regimens tailored to the number of risk factors present.[19]

Postoperative considerations include early resumption of normal diet, early ambulation, removal of catheters or drains as soon as possible, incorporation of epidural analgesia, use of defined discharge criteria, and continued goal-directed fluid, nausea, and opioid-sparing pain management.[2] Consuming a normal diet promotes early mobilization, supplies nutrients to muscles, reduces gastric dysmotility problems associated with surgery, and prevents stress-related ulcers. Defined discharge criteria include reaching milestones such as tolerating an oral diet, not requiring intravenous analgesics, ambulation, and having bowel movements. Further research has examined ERAS applications for various types of surgeries, such as esophageal, bariatric, orthopedic, gynecologic, and thoracic procedures.

ENHANCED RECOVERY AFTER SURGERY IN THE GERIATRIC POPULATION

Many studies have demonstrated comparable efficacy of implementing ERAS on surgical outcomes in both younger and geriatric patient populations. Baek and colleagues[20] prospectively evaluated 87 subjects older than age 70 years and 250 subjects younger than 70 years undergoing laparoscopic colorectal surgery with an ERAS fast-track program from 2009 to 2011. The older group was significantly more ill than the younger group as classified by the American Society of Anesthesiologists (ASA) physical status score (I:II:III, 33.8:57.1:9.1 vs 60.6:33.3:6.2%, respectively, P<.001), yet the postoperative course showed no differences in return of flatus, bowel movements, advancement of diet, removal of urinary catheter, complications, or length of postoperative stay. However, the older cohort did have more frequent visits to the emergency department and readmission within 1 month (11.7% vs 4%, P = .013). A systematic review by Bagnall and colleagues[21] evaluated 16 studies comparing ERAS care, in both elderly (age >75 years) and younger subject cohorts, to traditional care with respect to outcomes. Elderly subjects undergoing ERAS care had shorter hospital stays compared with elderly subjects with non-ERAS care (2 randomized controlled trials: 9 vs 13.2 days, respectively, P<.001; and 5.5 vs 7 days, respectively, P<.0001). These trials also revealed fewer complications associated with ERAS® protocols (27.4% vs 58.6%, P<.0001; and 5% vs 21.1%, P = .045). Most studies reviewed showed no differences in outcome between the older and younger groups in terms of hospital length of stay, morbidity, and mortality. Kisialeuski and colleagues[22] evaluated ERAS® protocol implementation after laparoscopic colorectal surgery in elderly subjects. Ninety-two subjects were divided into an older group (age >65 years) and a younger group. The older group had higher ASA scores but the study investigators found no difference in oral fluid tolerance (on day of surgery), first stool passage time, length of hospital stay, or number of perioperative complications. Slieker and colleagues[23] found no differences in urinary retention or postoperative ileus between older (age >70 years) and younger colorectal subjects undergoing ERAS-based care, even though Foley catheters and gastric tubes were present for a longer duration. The investigators also found that adherence to the ERAS pathway was comparable in the older and younger cohorts.

Wang and colleagues[24] evaluated the efficacy of ERAS-protocolized care after laparoscopic colorectal cancer resection in subjects older than the age of 65 years. The ERAS, or fast-track, protocol involved no preoperative bowel preparation, early postoperative oral diet, and earlier postoperative ambulation than the conventional perioperative care group. The fast-track group experienced shorter times to regain bowel function, to first bowel movement, and to start a liquid diet; reduced duration of postoperative hospital stay (P = .0001); and fewer complications (5.0% vs 21.1%, P = .045). Verheijen and colleagues[25] analyzed 348 subjects who underwent colorectal surgery from July 2006 to April 2008 and found that fast-track care can be implemented with a low complication rate in all subject groups, except that the length of stay in elderly subjects (age >80 years) averages 10 days versus 7 days in the younger group. Subjects undergoing emergency surgery also had longer lengths of stay (14 days), although the complication rates were comparably low, and goals of early initiation of enteral nutrition and early mobilization were equally feasible.

Jia and colleagues[26] evaluated a total of 240 elderly subjects (age 70–88 years) with colorectal carcinoma undergoing open surgery and randomly assigned subjects to either a traditional or ERAS-based fast-track care plan. In addition to evaluating the length of hospital stay and time to passing flatus, the group also assessed the incidence of postoperative delirium, a complication uniquely more prevalent in the elderly (subjects with a history of dementia, Parkinson disease, chronic alcohol abuse, sleeping pill or anxiolytic use, or who had received anesthesia within 30 days were excluded). The Delirium Rating Scale-Revised-98 (DRS-R-98) was used to evaluate mental status and cognitive function. It analyzes attention, orientation, and short-term and long-term memory, as well as visuospatial ability.[27] The DRS-R-98 was conducted on admission and up to postoperative day 5. The length of stay and time to pass flatus were shorter in the ERAS group (9.01 vs 13.21 days, respectively, $P<.001$; and 48.50 vs 77.66 hours, respectively, $P<.001$). More importantly, the incidence of postoperative delirium was significantly lower in the ERAS subjects (3.4% vs 12.9%, $P = .008$). The lower incidence of delirium was attributed to a statistically significant reduction in the serum levels of interleukin (IL)-6, which contributes to a systemic inflammatory response state.[28] Most incidents of postoperative delirium were diagnosed on postoperative days 1 and 2 for both groups and, interestingly, the serum IL-6 level also peaked in the immediate postoperative period on day 1 for both groups. Serum levels of IL-6 were significantly higher in the traditional group compared with the ERAS group at postoperative days 1 to 3. MRI scans were conducted for those with postoperative delirium and ruled out other causes of altered mental status, such as cerebral infarction or ischemia. Nursing care and haloperidol administered intramuscularly were used to treat delirium episodes. The investigators surmised that the incorporation of earlier oral feeding, the lack of use of mechanical enema and nasogastric tubes, and overall enhanced mobility could have curbed the stress inflammatory response in the ERAS group and hence reduced the incidence of postoperative delirium. Using fewer opioids and incorporating epidural anesthesia or analgesia (hindering the sympathetic response to pain) rather than general anesthesia also likely contributed to less delirium events.

The application of ERAS principles to geriatric subjects (age >70 years) after pancreaticoduodenectomy was evaluated by Partelli and colleagues[29] in a retrospective cohort study. The investigators used a 3:1 case-matched study protocol to compare 22 geriatric subjects receiving ERAS care to a matched group of 66 geriatric subjects receiving traditional care. Adherence to the ERAS® protocol was most difficult in 2 scenarios: starting a regular or solid diet by postoperative day 4 and removing surgical drains early. The investigators essentially demonstrated that an ERAS program for elderly subjects undergoing pancreaticoduodenectomy can be implemented in a safe manner because there was no difference in the rates of postoperative complications, readmissions, mortality rates, or reoperation rates. Of note, the overall length of stay was similar between the 2 groups, which could potentially be explained by the shorter than expected postoperative stay in the control group.

ENHANCED RECOVERY AFTER SURGERY IN THE EMERGENCY SURGERY AND TRAUMA POPULATIONS

As mentioned, prolonged hospital stays in the emergency surgery population are unavoidable due to the inherent nature of the sicker patient population often requiring multiple, repeated surgical interventions.[25] In addition, many preoperative and intraoperative ERAS considerations are not entirely feasible for implementation in the emergency timeframe, including preadmission education, early discharge planning, carbohydrate loading, reducing duration of fasting or nothing by mouth, incorporating minimally invasive surgery, and avoidance of drains. However, given the high rates of mortality associated with emergency surgeries (up to 80%), physicians are driving the use of ERAS principles in this population to potentially improve outcomes (**Fig. 2**).[30,31]

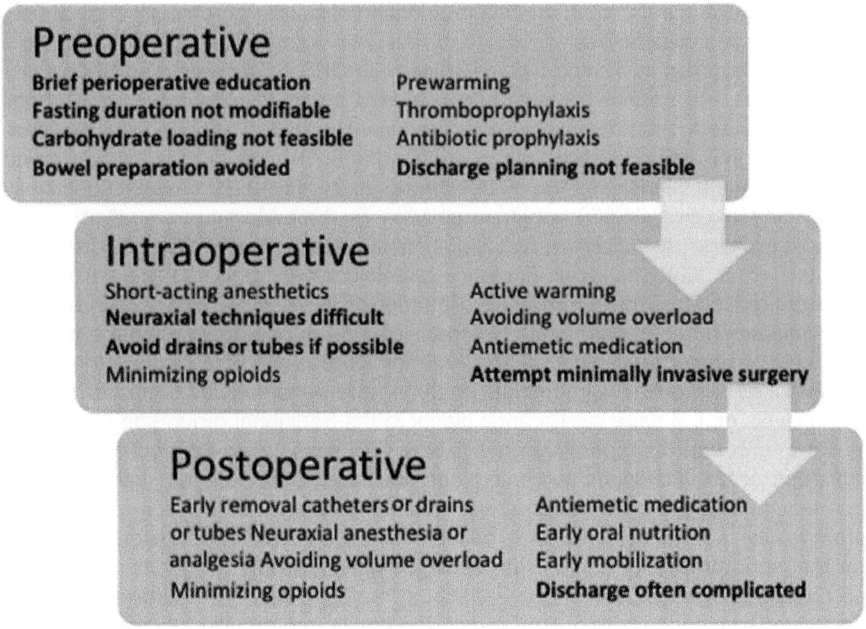

Preoperative

Brief perioperative education
Fasting duration not modifiable
Carbohydrate loading not feasible
Bowel preparation avoided

Prewarming
Thromboprophylaxis
Antibiotic prophylaxis
Discharge planning not feasible

Intraoperative

Short-acting anesthetics
Neuraxial techniques difficult
Avoid drains or tubes if possible
Minimizing opioids

Active warming
Avoiding volume overload
Antiemetic medication
Attempt minimally invasive surgery

Postoperative

Early removal catheters or drains
or tubes Neuraxial anesthesia or
analgesia Avoiding volume overload
Minimizing opioids

Antiemetic medication
Early oral nutrition
Early mobilization
Discharge often complicated

Fig. 2. Acute care surgery ERAS® protocol.

Paduraru and colleagues[32] conducted a systematic review of using ERAS after emergency surgery and evaluated 4 cohort studies and 1 randomized controlled trial. The average number of ERAS items implemented was 11 to 18 of the recommended 20 by the ERAS® Society. Key results included fewer postoperative complications, shorter length of stay, and equal or reduced mortality in the ERAS intervention groups compared with conventional care groups. Overall, Paduraru and colleagues[32] noticed a reduced compliance rate to ERAS principles in the acute care setting, which called for greater education and adaptation of such management principles by the multidisciplinary staff taking care of these subjects.

Gonenc and colleagues[33] examined the implementation of ERAS principles in emergency laparoscopic surgery for perforated (less than 10 mm in size) peptic ulcer disease. Two subject groups (adult and geriatric population) were selected in a randomized fashion, with 1 receiving standardized postoperative care and the other receiving ERAS-protocolized care. Examples of interventions in the ERAS group included removal of the urinary catheter and nasogastric tube in the operating room immediately postoperatively (as opposed to later in the hospital stay when the drainage content became <300 mL per day), and administering liquids on postoperative day 1 and soft food on day 2 (vs after the passage of flatus or stool in the conventional group). The primary endpoints were length of stay and morbidity or mortality during the first 30 days after surgery. Length of stay was significantly shorter in the ERAS intervention group (3.8 vs 6.9 days, $P = .0001$). There was no statistically significant difference in morbidity or mortality between the 2 groups. Postoperative ileus was found less frequently in the ERAS group; this was attributed to the reduction in nasogastric decompression use, reduced opiate use, early enteral feeding, and the use of nonsteroidal antiinflammatory drugs for postoperative pain.

Lohsiriwat[34] evaluated the implementation of ERAS pathways after emergency colorectal surgery using case-matched cohorts at a single hospital from January 2011 to October 2013. Adult and geriatric subjects were matched by severity of illness and operative severity score, and primary outcomes included length of hospital stay and postoperative morbidity. A total of 20 subjects in the ERAS group were compared with 40 subjects receiving conventional care. Median hospital length of stay was shorter in the ERAS group (5.5 days, range 3–16 days, vs 7.5 days, range 5–25 days, $P = .009$). The ERAS group also had a shorter time to first flatus (1.6 days vs 2.8 days, $P<.001$) and reduced time to tolerating a regular diet (3.5 days vs 5.5 days, $P = .002$). The incidence of postoperative complications was less in the ERAS group (although nonsignificant), and the investigators found no increase in 30-day readmission even though the hospital length of stay was reduced. Limitations of the study include a small sample size and selection of low-risk subjects. The shorter time to passage of first flatus may be aided by restrictive intravenous fluid administration as well. ERAS® guidelines recommend the use of warmed intravenous fluids, and favor boluses with colloid or crystalloid rather than continuous infusions for mainte-nance.[6] This goal-directed fluid therapy strategy minimizes volume overload and sub-sequent complications, such as bowel edema and extravascular lung edema. Adjunctive use of vasopressors minimizes further superfluous fluid administration to offset the hypotensive effects of intraoperative anesthetic and analgesic medications, as well as epidural-induced sympathectomy.

Wisely and Barclay[35] conducted a retrospective multicenter cohort database study comparing adult and geriatric subjects undergoing emergency abdominal surgery from October 2008 and May 2010 with subjects undergoing similar surgery in the post-ERAS timeframe from January 2011 to December 2012. Examples of the most frequent operations include right-sided colon resections (22%), adhesiolysis (20%), and small bowel resections (22%), with obstruction being the most common emer-gency condition. The study included 370 subjects, and there were statistically signif-icant reductions in many post-ERAS variables, including reduced intraoperative fluid administration (from 2520 mL to 2000 mL, $P<.001$) and postoperative 48-hour total intravenous fluid administration (from 5382 mL to 2890 mL, $P<.001$). Significant reduc-tions in the use of a urinary catheter (57% vs 77%, $P<.001$), drain (43% vs 60%, $P = .001$), and opioid patient-controlled analgesia (20% vs 36%, $P = .001$) were found at 2 days postoperatively in the post-ERAS group. Fewer subjects in the post-ERAS group received total parenteral nutrition (18% vs 32%, $P = .001$). Significantly fewer major complications, such as acute renal failure, sepsis, intraabdominal infections, and small bowel obstruction, were found in the post-ERAS group, and this was signif-icantly related to 48-hour fluid balance. Additional complications, such as urinary tract infections, urinary retention, and respiratory infections, were all reduced to a signifi-cant extent in the post-ERAS group.

Roulin and colleagues[36] conducted a prospective cohort study evaluating adult and geriatric subjects undergoing urgent colectomies and treated with an ERAS® protocol between April 2012 and March 2013, and compared them to subjects undergoing elective colectomy with ERAS care. Twenty-eight subjects in the urgent colectomy group were compared with 63 subjects undergoing elective colectomy. ERAS® proto-col components included avoidance of bowel preparation; 2-hour and 6-hour fasting for liquids and solids, respectively; carbohydrate loading; minimal preoperative seda-tives; low-molecular weight heparin and antibiotic prophylaxis; epidural analgesia; postoperative nausea or vomiting prophylaxis; restrictive or balanced intravenous fluids; avoiding nasogastric tubes or abdominal drains; epidural removal after 48 hours; ambulation on the day of surgery; normal diet resumption on the day of surgery; laxative administration; and removal of the urinary catheter on postoperative day 1. Preoperative compliance with the ERAS® protocol was 64 versus 96% (P<.001) for the urgent and elective procedures, respectively; intraoperative compliance was 77 versus 86% (P = .145), respectively; and postoperative compliance was 49 versus 67% (P = .015), respectively. Difficult items to implement in the urgent surgery group included preadmission subject education (0%), preoperative carbohydrate drinks (25%), prophylactic antiemetics (39%), oral nutritional supplements on the day of surgery (39%), and removal of Foley catheter on day 1 (32%). Median postoperative length of stay was 8 days in the urgent setting compared with 5 days in the elective setting (P = .006). More cardiovascular events and pneumonia were seen in the urgent group (P = .010 and P = .027, respectively). Time to first bowel motion was similar in the 2 groups, with a median of 3 postoperative days. There was no increase in overall complication rates with the implementation of the ERAS® protocol in the urgent surgery group, even though this group had higher ASA and Portsmouth Physiologic and Operative Severity Score for the Enumeration of Mortality and Morbidity (P-POS-SUM) scores and had more open procedures, as well as ostomy creations.

Moydien and colleagues[37] conducted a single-center pilot study evaluating a prospective cohort of 38 subjects with isolated penetrating abdominal trauma requiring emergency laparotomy from January to December 2013. This group was compared with a historical group of 40 subjects who had undergone the same emergency surgery but without an ERAS recovery protocol. Both groups were similar in terms of age, gender, mechanism of injury, and time to laparotomy. The enhanced recovery protocols included early nasogastric tube removal, early feeding (solids and liquids), early urinary catheter removal, early mobilization, early removal of intravenous lines, and early transition from intravenous (morphine and acetaminophen over the first 48 hours) to oral analgesia. All subjects (including historical subjects) were mobilized on postoperative day 1 with the help of physical therapy. Primary endpoints included hospital length of stay and occurrence of postoperative complications. T-tests were used for the primary analysis. Subjects in the ERAS group had earlier removal of nasogastric tubes (1.2 vs 2.1 days, P<.0042), earlier removal of urinary catheters (1.9 vs 3.3 days, P<.00003), and less time to initiation of a solid diet (2.8 vs 3.6 days, P<.035). There was no statistically significant difference in postoperative complications between the 2 groups. Notably, the ERAS group had a significantly shorter mean hospital length of stay (5.5 vs 8.4 days, P<.00021).

SUMMARY

The incorporation of ERAS fundamentals into perioperative medicine has improved the patient care experience and hastened recovery time while reducing hospital costs.[5] Incorporating ERAS principles in the adult or geriatric acute care surgery patient populations has been shown to minimize time to resumption of preoperative activity in addition to reducing hospital length of stay. Elderly patients had lower incidence rates of delirium when patient care was focused on decreasing the time to resumption of normal diet and activity while minimizing the use of drains and invasive tubes; the addition of routine geriatric consults to this population may increase the number of formal cognitive evaluations and improve advanced care planning.[38] The application of ERAS in trauma patients seems promising based on limited evidence. These unique emergency surgery patient populations benefit from ERAS® protocols using decreased opioids and decreased intravenous fluids while enduring no major setbacks in terms of morbidity and mortality. ERAS principles are widely applicable to these patient populations, and increased physician and nursing training to promote widespread utilization of ERAS® protocols will further improve quality of health care administered in the twenty-first century.

REFERENCES

1. Pędziwiatr M, Mavrikis J, Witowski J, et al. Current status of enhanced recovery after surgery (ERAS) protocol in gastrointestinal surgery. Med Oncol 2018; 35(6):95.
2. Ljungqvist O, Scott M, Fearon KC. Enhanced recovery after surgery: a review. JAMA Surg 2017;152:292–8.
3. Gustafsson UO, Scott MJ, Schwenk W, et al. Guidelines for perioperative care in elective colonic surgery: Enhanced Recovery After Surgery (ERAS®) Society recommendations. Clin Nutr 2012;31(6):783–800.
4. Nygren J, Thacker J, Carli F, et al. Guidelines for perioperative care in elective rectal/pelvic surgery: Enhanced Recovery After Surgery (ERAS®) Society recommendations. Clin Nutr 2012;31(6):801–16.
5. Lassen K, Coolsen MM, Slim K, et al. Guidelines for perioperative care for pancreaticoduodenectomy: Enhanced Recovery After Surgery (ERAS®) Society recommendations. Clin Nutr 2012;31(6):817–30.
6. Lassen K, Soop M, Nygren J, et al. Consensus review of optimal perioperative care in colorectal surgery: Enhanced Recovery After Surgery (ERAS) Group recommendations. Arch Surg 2009;144:961–9.
7. Raghunathan K, Singh M, Lobo DN. Fluid management in abdominal surgery: what, when, and when not to administer. Anesthesiol Clin 2015;33(1):51–64.
8. Melnyk M, Casey RG, Black P, et al. Enhanced recovery after surgery (ERAS®) protocols: time to change practice? Can Urol Assoc J 2011;5:342–8.
9. Pędziwiatr M, Wierdak M, Nowakowski M, et al. Cost minimization analysis of laparoscopic surgery for colorectal cancer within the enhanced recovery after surgery (ERAS) protocol: a single-centre, case-matched study. Wideochir Inne Tech Maloinwazyjne 2016;11:14–21.
10. Kingsnorth A, Bowley D. Fundamentals of surgical practice: a preparation guide for the intercollegiate MRCS examination. 3rd edition. New York: Cambridge University Press; 2011. p. 181–9.
11. Brady M, Kinn S, Stuart P. Preoperative fasting for adults to prevent perioperative complications. Cochrane Database Syst Rev 2003;(4):CD004423.
12. Awad S, Varadhan KK, Ljungqvist O, et al. A meta-analysis of randomised controlled trials on preoperative oral carbohydrate treatment in elective surgery. Clin Nutr 2013;32(1):34–44.
13. Holte K, Nielsen KG, Madsen JL, et al. Physiologic effects of bowel preparation. Dis Colon Rectum 2004;47:1397–402.
14. Bucher P, Mermillod B, Gervaz P, et al. Mechanical bowel preparation for elective colorectal surgery: a meta-analysis. Arch Surg 2004;139(12):1359–65.
15. Fearon KCH, Ljungqvist O, Von Meyenfeldt M, et al. Enhanced recovery after surgery: a consensus review of clinical care for patients undergoing colonic resection. Clin Nutr 2005;24:466–77.
16. Hannemann P, Lassen K, Hausel J, et al. Patterns in current anaesthesiological peri-operative practice for colonic resections: a survey in five northern-European countries. Acta Anaesthesiol Scand 2006;50(9):1152–60.
17. Lobo DN, Bostock KA, Neal KR, et al. Effect of salt and water balance on recovery of gastrointestinal function after elective colonic resection: a randomized controlled trial. Lancet 2002;359:1812–8.

18. Lobo DN, Macafee DA, Allison SP. How perioperative fluid balance influences postoperative outcomes. Best Pract Res Clin Anaesthesiol 2006;20:439–55.
19. Leslie K, Myles PS, Chan MT, et al. Risk factors for severe postoperative nausea and vomiting in a randomized trial of nitrous oxide-based vs nitrous oxide-free anaesthesia. Br J Anaesth 2008;101(4):498–505.
20. Baek S-J, Kim S-H, Kim S-Y, et al. The safety of a "fast-track" program after laparoscopic colorectal surgery is comparable in older patients as in younger patients. Surg Endosc 2013;27:1225–32.
21. Bagnall NM, Malietzis G, Kennedy RH, et al. A systematic review of enhanced recovery care after colorectal surgery in elderly patients. Colorectal Dis 2014;16: 947–56.
22. Kisialeuski M, Pędziwiatr M, Matłok M, et al. Enhanced recovery after colorectal surgery in elderly patients. Wideochir Inne Tech Maloinwazyjne 2015;10:30–6.
23. Slieker J, Frauche P, Jurt J, et al. Enhanced recovery ERAS for elderly: a safe and beneficial pathway in colorectal surgery. Int J Colorectal Dis 2017;32:215–21.
24. Wang Q, Suo J, Jiang J, et al. Effectiveness of fast-track rehabilitation vs conventional care in laparoscopic colorectal resection for elderly patients: a randomized trial. Colorectal Dis 2012;14:1009–13.
25. Verheijen PM, Vd Ven AWH, Davids PHP, et al. Feasibility of enhanced recovery programme in various patient groups. Int J Colorectal Dis 2012;27:507–11.
26. Jia Y, Jin G, Guo S, et al. Fast-track surgery decreases the incidence of postoperative delirium and other complications in elderly patients with colorectal carcinoma. Langenbecks Arch Surg 2014;399(1):77–84.
27. Trzepacz PT, Mittal D, Torres R, et al. Validation of the Delirium Rating Scale-revised-98: comparison with the delirium rating scale and the cognitive test for delirium. J Neuropsychiatry Clin Neurosci 2001;13(2):229–42.
28. Holmes C, Cunningham C, Zotova E, et al. Proinflammatory cytokines, sickness behavior, and Alzheimer disease. Neurology 2011;77:212–8.
29. Partelli S, Crippa S, Castagnani R, et al. Evaluation of an enhanced recovery protocol after pancreaticoduodenectomy in elderly patients. HPB (Oxford) 2016; 18(2):153–8.
30. Emergency surgery. Emergency surgery policy briefing. Royal college of surgeons. 2014. Available at: https://www.rcseng.ac.uk/-/media/files/rcs/about-rcs/government-relations-consultation/rcs-emergency-surgery-policy-briefing. pdf. Accessed July 30, 2018.
31. Iain A. The future of emergency general surgery: a joint document. Association of Coloproctology of Great Britain and Ireland, Association of Upper Gastro-intestinal Surgeons & Association of Surgeons of Great Britain and Ireland. 2015. Available at: http://www.augis.org/wp-content/uploads/2014/05/Future-of-EGSjoint-document_Iain-Anderson_140915.pdf. Accessed July 30, 2018.
32. Paduraru M, Ponchietti L, Casas IM, et al. Enhanced recovery after emergency surgery: a systematic review. Bull Emerg Trauma 2017;5(2):70–8.
33. Gonenc M, Dural AC, Celik F, et al. Enhanced postoperative recovery pathways in emergency surgery: a randomised controlled clinical trial. Am J Surg 2014; 207(6):807–14.
34. Lohsiriwat V. Enhanced recovery after surgery vs conventional care in emergency colorectal surgery. World J Gastroenterol 2014;20(38):13950–5.
35. Wisely JC, Barclay KL. Effects of an enhanced recovery after surgery programme on emergency surgical patients. ANZ J Surg 2016;86(11):883–8.
36. Roulin D, Blanc C, Muradbegovic M, et al. Enhanced recovery pathway for urgent colectomy. World J Surg 2014;38(8):2153–9.

37. Moydien MR, Oodit R, Chowdhury S, et al. Enhanced recovery after surgery (ERAS) in penetrating abdominal trauma: a prospective single-center pilot study. S Afr J Surg 2016;54(4):7–10.
38. Olufajo OA, Tulebaev S, Javedan H, et al. Integrating geriatric consults into routine care of older trauma patients: one-year experience of a level 1 trauma center. J Am Coll Surg 2016;222(6):1029–35.

Pain Management in Trauma in the Age of the Opioid Crisis

Jessica Lynn Gross, MD[a], Alison R. Perate, MD[b],
Nabil M. Elkassabany, MD, MSCE[c],*

KEYWORDS

- Pain management • Opioids • Opioid crisis • Multimodal pain analgesia
- Adult trauma • Pediatric trauma

KEY POINTS

- Multimodality pain therapies that include using acetaminophen, nonsteroidal antiinflammatory drugs, and/or gabapentin have been demonstrated to have opioid-sparing effects.
- Pain management goals should include adequately treating pain with the least amount of opioids to decrease the chance for dependence and/or overdose.
- Minimizing exposure of children to opioids plays an important role in combatting the current opioid crisis.
- Standardized pain management protocols may reduce opioid use while maintaining pain control and patient satisfaction.

We need to train doctors and nurses to treat pain as a vital sign. Quality care means that pain is measured. Quality of care means that pain is treated...That is, that proper assessment and treatment of pain in the hospital will become part of the standard of care that hospitals must provide.[1]
—*Dr. James N. Campbell during his 1995 Presidential Address to the American Pain Society[1]*

PAIN MANAGEMENT IN ADULT TRAUMA

In 2001, The Joint Commission set pain standards for health care organizations in response to the national outcry that pain is undertreated.[2] The Joint Commission

Disclosures: The authors have nothing to disclose.
[a] Wake Forest School of Medicine, Wake Forest Baptist Medical Center, Medical Center Boulevard, Winston Salem, NC 27157, USA; [b] Department of Anesthesiology and Critical Care, The Children's Hospital of Philadelphia, Perelman School of Medicine, University of Pennsylvania, 3401 Civic Center Boulevard, Philadelphia, PA 19104, USA; [c] Department of Anesthesiology and Critical Care, Perelman School of Medicine, University of Pennsylvania, 3400 Spruce Street, Dulles 6, Philadelphia, PA 19104, USA
* Corresponding author.
E-mail address: Nabil.Elkassabany@uphs.upenn.edu

Anesthesiology Clin 37 (2019) 79–91
https://doi.org/10.1016/j.anclin.2018.09.010
1932-2275/19/© 2018 Elsevier Inc. All rights reserved.

anesthesiology.theclinics.com

Comprehensive Accreditation Manual for Hospitals highlighted the importance of early pain management for trauma patients.[3] Furthermore, they emphasized that all patients must receive appropriate pain control regimens and provided the following standards:

1. Patients should have an initial assessment of pain followed by serial reassessments of pain.
2. All relevant providers should be educated on pain assessment and pain management.
3. The patients and their families (when appropriate) should be educated on their roles in pain management, the potential limitations of pain control therapies, and the side effects of pain medications.
4. Communicating to patients and families that pain management is an important part of their medical care.

Health care organizations were also encouraged to use pain scales, such as the numeric rating scale (range 0–10), the verbal rating scale, or the Wong-Baker FACES Pain Rating Scale (cartoons of smiling to grimacing faces), to assess the severity of pain.[2] Quality improvement initiatives were implemented to assess the adequacy of pain control management provided by health care providers. One such initiative evaluated the quality of pain control provided by health care organizations through postdischarge surveys sent to patients. The surveys included the following questions:

1. Need medicine for pain? (yes or no)
2. Pain well-controlled? (never, sometimes, usually, or always)
3. Staff did everything to help with pain? (never, sometimes, usually, or always).[4]

The survey results were used to calculate the Patient Experience of Care Domain score of the Hospital Consumer Assessment of Healthcare Providers and Systems (HCAHPS). Overall, the HCAHPS score is used as part of the Hospital Value-Based Purchasing program. Similarly, the Centers for Medicare and Medicaid Services developed a quality measure of pain management by assessing the time it took for long-bone fracture patients to receive pain medication after emergency room arrival.[5] Decreased HCAHPS scores may result in lower reimbursement rates from health care insurance companies. Providing high-quality pain control can be challenging, especially in the setting of the current opioid abuse epidemic.[6] There is an ongoing debate about whether the addition of these subjective questions to the postdischarge survey may have contributed to the increase in opioid prescriptions.

Although pain is not unidimensional, patients are often asked to measure their level of pain on a numeric scale.[2] Cepeda and colleagues conducted a study on 700 adult subjects who were asked to rate their pain using numeric scale and then indicate the degree of pain improvement after each pain intervention on a 5-point Likert scale (ranging from no improvement to complete pain relief). A decrease of 1.3 units was associated with minimal improvement, a decrease of 2.4 units was associated with much improvement, and a decrease of 3.5 units was associated with very much improvement in pain.[7] The results demonstrated that a subject's perception of pain reduction parallels a decrease in pain intensity along a numerical scale. Investigators also found that the change in pain intensity that is meaningful to a subject increases as the severity of his or her baseline pain increases.[7] This study suggests that the numerical scale is a reasonable assessment of a patient's pain and response to pain medication.

Physiologically, postoperative or posttrauma pain involves the activation of different pain pathways, including nociceptive, neuropathic, and inflammatory mechanisms.[8] Nociceptive pain is produced by noxious stimuli. Opioids are often used to address nociceptive pain. As with all medications, opioids are associated with several risks and benefits. The benefits of acute pain relief are clear; however, the risks of opioid medications vary widely and include hyperalgesia, oversedation, nausea, vomiting, ileus, respiratory depression, risk for overdose, withdrawal after prolonged use, nonmedical use, abuse, addiction, and death.[9] Neuropathic pain is described as "pain arising as a direct consequence of a lesion or disease affecting the somatosensory system."[10] Treating neuropathic pain is a challenge because many report pain that is refractory to traditional pharmacotherapy. Medications such as tricyclic antidepressants, selective serotonin norepinephrine reuptake inhibitors, and calcium channel α-δ ligand (ie, gabapentin or pregabalin) are considered first-line for treatment of neuropathic pain. Tramadol and opioid analgesics are second-line treatments.[10] Gabapentin, which was introduced as an antiepileptic in 1993, has been used extensively to treat neuropathic pain. Gabapentin (and pregabalin) are believed to bind to the 21 subunits of the presynaptic voltage-gated calcium channels, which are upregulated in the dorsal root ganglia and spinal cord after surgical trauma. By blocking the influx of calcium via these channels, the release of excitatory neurotransmitters is inhibited. This allows gabapentin to have antiallodynic and antihyperanalgesic properties with only minimal effects on normal nociception.[11] The inflammatory process around the affected area results in hypersensitivity to pain in that area. Prostaglandin production reduces the threshold for activation and increases the responsiveness of nociceptive terminals. Cyclooxgenase-2 (COX-2) inhibitors and nonsteroidal antiinflammatory drugs (NSAIDs) prevent the conversion of arachidonic acid to prostaglandin H.[12]

Every day, more than 115 Americans die from opioid overdose.[13] Prescription opioids account for approximately 70% of fatal prescription drug overdoses.[14] Therefore, the nonmedical use of opioids is a major health problem.[15] The Centers for Disease Control and Prevention estimates that the total economic burden of prescription opioid overdose, abuse, and dependence (ie, health care costs, lost productivity, additional treatment, and criminal justice) was around 78.5 billion dollars in 2013.[14] This stems from increasing numbers of emergency room visits, hospital admissions, and fatal overdoses from prescription opioids.[15] The amount of opioid prescriptions has been increasing over time. For example, opioid prescriptions in 1997 were calculated to be 96 morphine milligram equivalents (MME) per person. This number escalated to 700 MME per person in 2007. The 700 MME would allow every adult American to have a 3-week supply of 5 mg hydrocodone if taken every 4 hours.[16] By 2010, enough opioid pain relievers were prescribed to expand the duration to a 4-eek supply.[17] Some providers believe it was the addition of the pain management questions in the HCAHPS surveys that lead to the increase in opioid prescriptions; however, data from the National Institute on Drug Abuse demonstrated that there was already an increase in opioid prescription before the implementation of The Joint Commission's new pain standards.[18]

Opioids are commonly prescribed for injury and after surgical procedures. A systematic review of 810 subjects who underwent various surgical procedures demonstrated that 67% to 92% reported having unused opioids. Subjects reported ranges of 42% to 71% of unused opioid tablets. Most subjects, 71% to 83%, stopped using opioids due to adequate pain control. Of these unused tablets, only 4% to 30% subjects planned to or actually disposed of their unused opioids. Of these individuals, only 4% to 9% considered or used a disposal method recommended by the US Food and Drug Administration (FDA).[19] These numbers imply that most patients do not need all of the opioid medication that are prescribed. The reported low pill disposal rate suggests that these opioids remain in the community.

It has been suggested that prescription opioids are the drug of choice for abuse for various reasons. These reasons include that they are easier to obtain than illicit drugs; purchasing illicit drugs is monitored by law enforcement, making arrests more likely; the use or abuse of prescriptions drugs is more socially acceptable, and the purity of prescription drugs is more reliable and, thus, theoretically safer than illicit drugs.[20] It is important for physicians to recognize individuals who are misusing and/or abusing opioids. Thirty-six percent of individuals who misused opioids obtained a prescription from 1 or more physicians. Additionally, more than half of the people (54%) who misused prescription opioids obtained the drug from a friend or relative,[19] which poses the question: are health care providers overprescribing opioids and contributing to the opioid abuse epidemic?

Webster and Webster[21] developed and studied an opioid risk tool (ORT) to identify patients at high risk for opioid misuse or abuse. The ORT was administered to new patients presenting to the pain clinic (**Table 1**). Each risk factor was weighted based on the physician's own clinical experience and review of the literature. These weights were created before the start of the study and were not modified during the study. The tool is a point-based system (minimum 0, maximum 26). On completion of the ORT survey, subjects were divided into 3 groups based on their likelihood to abuse opioids. Scoring was as follows: low risk (0–3); moderate risk (4–7), and high risk (>8). The subjects were then observed over a 12-month period to see if they displayed any aberrant behaviors such as using more opioids than prescribed, selling prescriptions, positive blood or urine drug screen, resistance to changes in therapy, reporting lost or stolen prescriptions, and/or requesting early refills. At the conclusion of the study, 37 out of 108 women and 39 out of 77 men displayed 1 or more aberrant behaviors. Of those who scored as low risk on ORT (18 subjects), only 1 subject displayed aberrant behaviors. For those who scored as moderate risk (123 subjects),

Table 1
Opioid risk tool

Item	Mark Each Box That Applies	Item Score if Female	Item Score if Male
Family history			
Alcohol		1	3
Illegal drugs		2	3
Prescription drugs		4	4
Personal history			
Alcohol		3	3
Illegal drugs		4	4
Prescription drugs		5	5
Age between 16 and 45 years		1	1
History of preadolescent sexual abuse		3	0
Psychological disease			
(Attention-deficit hyperactivity disorder, obsessive-compulsive disorder, bipolar, or schizophrenia)		2	2
Depression		1	1
Total score			

Adapted from Webster LR, Webster RM. Predicting aberrant behaviors in opioid-treated patients: preliminary validation of the opioid risk tool. Pain Med 2005;6(6):433; with permission.

only 35 displayed aberrant behaviors; thus, they were 2.5 times more likely to not abuse opioids than to abuse opioids. For those who scored as high risk, 40 out of 44 displayed aberrant behaviors, indicating that those who score as high risk are likely to abuse or misuse opioids. These data suggest that a high score on the ORT is a risk factor for abusing or misusing opioids, and that physicians should proceed with caution when prescribing opioids to these individuals.

In 2011, the US Office of National Drug Control policy issued recommendations for all states to have prescription drug-monitoring programs (PDMPs).[14] It was believed that the creation of PDMPs would decrease the number of opioid overdoses because 40% of subjects who had drug overdoses received prescriptions for high-dose opioids from multiple physicians. Twenty percent of these overdoses occurred in individuals with low-dose opioid prescriptions (<100 MME/d) given by a single provider. Forty percent of the prescription overdoses occurred in individuals receiving greater than 100 MME per day by a single provider.[17] These monitoring systems enabled physicians to see an individual's opioid prescriptions history. As of 2018, 49 states, the District of Columbia, and 1 US territory (Guam) have operational PDMPs. Missouri is the only state that currently does not have a statewide PDMP; however, St. Louis County implemented a PDMP that serves more than half of the population of Missouri.[22]

The Researched Abuse, Diversion, and Addiction-Related Surveillance (RADARS) system is a prescription drug abuse, misuse, and diversion surveillance system with 6 unique programs that collect prescription opioid and stimulant drug data from different target populations and report this data on a quarterly basis. Reifler and colleagues[23] used data from the RADARS System Poison Center and Opioid Treatment to evaluate the efficacy of PDMPs on opioid abuse and misuse patterns. The date of enactment of each state's prescription monitoring program was obtained and the states were divided into 3 groups: no active PDMP before or during the surveillance period, PDMP implemented before surveillance period, or PDMP implemented during the surveillance period. Implementation was defined as when the PDMP began collecting prescription data. The study reported an association between having a PDMP and a decrease in opioid abuse and misuse, as well as lower opioid treatment admissions. Although larger scale studies are required, the initial results from this study suggest that PDMPs may be effective in mitigating the effects of the opioid abuse crisis.

Pain is a subjective experience and depends on a variety of biological, psychological, and social factors.[24] Unfortunately, less than half of US patients who undergo surgery report adequate pain relief.[25] Additionally, substance and opioid abuse disorders are prevalent in a large proportion of trauma patients who may require substantially higher opioid medication dosages and may be more likely to report unsatisfactory pain control.[26,27] Undertreatment of acute pain may be associated with adverse consequences, including pneumonia, decreased mobilization, deep venous thrombosis or pulmonary emboli, hindered recovery, and/or progression to chronic pain. This may ultimately affect a patient's physical rehabilitation process, ability to perform functions of daily living, workforce performance, and ability to return to a job. The patient may then develop psychological disorders, such as anxiety or depression. All of these may lead to significant health care costs and/or need for disability.[28] It is important that pain is not only assessed when the patient is at rest but also when participating in physical or occupational therapy.[25] To provide the most effective pain control, it is imperative that a provider accurately measure a patient's degree of pain, address the multiple factors that affect the patient's pain, and use multimodality pain regimens (increasing the use of nonopioid medications) to treat pain through its numerous pathways and receptors.[8]

Regional anesthesia and analgesia can potentially be integrated into a multimodal analgesia protocol for acute trauma patients, especially for long bone fractures. The widespread use of ultrasound and the abundance of educational materials have made learning and successfully performing peripheral nerve blockade (PNB) more accessible. The military has successfully used PNB, often in austere environments, to not only deliver targeted analgesia to enable surgical interventions but also as part of pain management protocols after acute trauma. Advantages of using PNB for analgesia include preserving airway patency, mental status, and hemodynamics.[29] Many civilian trauma centers are offering PNBs in the prehospital and emergency department as part of acute pain management models.[30] Multiple studies have demonstrated the benefits of PNBs (eg, femoral nerve block, fascia iliaca block) used to manage perioperative pain associated with hip fractures.[31–33] Furthermore, PNB catheters can be placed to provide pain relief over the course of several days. Neuraxial anesthesia (ie, epidural catheter) is also crucial in the treatment of perioperative pain and, barring any contraindications, was considered to be a level I recommendation in the management of traumatic rib fractures per the 2005 Eastern Association for the Surgery of Trauma (EAST) practice guidelines.[34] However, recent studies have challenged this recommendation because they reported an association between epidural analgesia and increased respiratory complications and hospital length of stay.[35] The most recent 2016 joint recommendations published by EAST and the Trauma Anesthesiology Society have downgraded their recommendation of epidural analgesia use in blunt thoracic adult trauma to conditional use in conjunction with multimodal analgesia; they do still maintain that opioids should not be used as the sole therapy to manage blunt thoracic trauma pain. Additionally, these recommendations are based on very low-quality studies and scarce data regarding the optimal pain management strategies in this patient population.[36] Truncal blocks (ie, ultrasound-guided paravertebral, intercostal, serratus anterior plane, and erector spinae plane blocks) are alternatives to traditional neuraxial analgesic techniques.[37–39] However, provider inexperience, prioritizing resuscitation, and concerns for masking acute compartment syndrome,[40] in addition to other regional block side effects (eg, local anesthetic systemic toxicity, postblock nerve injuries, bleeding), are often cited as reasons for limiting regional anesthesia use in the acute trauma setting.[41]

The current emphasis on pain management strategies is to use a multimodal approach to decrease opioid use. Acetaminophen, a nonopioid analgesic, has been shown to be opioid-sparing. Randomized controlled trials demonstrated that the addition of acetaminophen significantly reduces 24-hour morphine consumption.[42] The decrease in opioid consumption was not only demonstrated with concurrent acetaminophen use (mean reduction of morphine dose of 6.34 mg), but also with NSAIDS (10.18 mg reduction), and COX-2 inhibitors (10.92 mg reduction). In fact, NSAIDs and COX-2 inhibitors have a statistically significant greater decrease in morphine consumption compared with acetaminophen.[43] Preoperative administration of celecoxib was also demonstrated to decrease opioid use and was associated with lower postoperative pain scores.[25] Furthermore, agents such as gabapentin, when given as a single preoperative dose, demonstrated a reduction in opioid analgesic requirements and pain scores during the first postoperative 24-hours without major adverse effects, after different surgeries. The opioid-sparing effect was not associated with the gabapentin dosage.[11]

In trauma patients, there is a concern for providers writing excessive amounts of opioid prescriptions on discharge. At Wake Forest Baptist Medical Center, a multidisciplinary team, made up of members from the departments of trauma and orthopedic surgery, anesthesiology (both acute and chronic pain providers), psychiatry, and pharmacy, was created to gain better insight into the pain management and prescription practices in trauma patients. The team identified 3 specific weaknesses in the management of pain in the trauma services: (1) the lack of a standardized approach to inpatient pain management, (2) the lack of standardized weaning process for those discharged on opioid medications, and (3) the lack of education for both patients and providers about opioid use. They created a pain management protocol that standardized pain control in a step-wise fashion (**Fig. 1**). They also provided the patients with a wean plan in their discharge instructions, along with educational materials on opioids. This standardized trauma patient pain management strategy demonstrated a statistically significant decrease in MME in the outpatient setting while maintaining overall patient satisfaction and pain control.[44] Further studies evaluating such standardized trauma pain management protocols are required. It is important that the protocols should be tailored to each individual institution based on available resources and needs.

PAIN MANAGEMENT IN PEDIATRIC TRAUMA

Trauma is the leading cause of morbidity and mortality in the pediatric population in the United States,[45] with approximately 10 million children annually presenting with traumatic injuries.[46] Many of these pediatric trauma patients sustain injuries that cause life-long disability. To minimize the severity and duration of the traumatic injuries, both the acute and chronic pain must be treated effectively. Ascending nociceptive neural pathways develop by 23-week gestation in the fetus.[47] Painful stimuli result in stress reactions that may lead to neuroapoptosis, decreased brain growth, and neurocognitive impairments later in life.[48] Children are most vulnerable to the adverse effects of pain during the formation of these neural synapses.[49] Infants and young children also have a lower threshold for stimulation of nociceptive receptors, which may lead to hyperalgesia.[50] For these reasons, adequate treatment of pain is important not only to provide comfort in the acute setting but also to minimize long-term sequelae from injury.

Over the last decade, new pediatric pain assessment scales have been developed and validated, resulting in a systematic approach to evaluating and responding to pediatric pain.[51] With standardized measuring tools, pediatric pain management moved to evidence-based protocols. Although randomized controlled trials assessing nonopioid techniques are lacking in the pediatric trauma population, the use of multimodal or

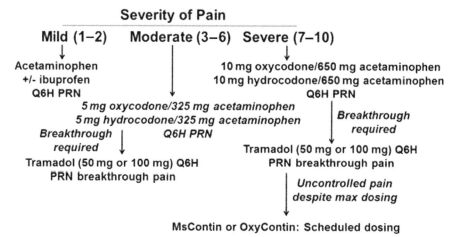

Fig. 1. Pain management protocol.

balanced technique pain management strategies are encouraged.[52] In the pediatric population, almost 5% of patients have persistent opioid use after surgery.[53] Using pain management plans in pediatric trauma patients that use an armamentarium of different classes of nonopioid medications may help reduce opioid use and may play a crucial role in combatting the current national opioid crisis. A multimodal approach using nonopioid oral and intravenous (IV) medications and nerve blocks is preferred in the pediatric population.[54,55] Historically, local anesthetic infiltration has been used in the pediatric population for various injuries with successful reduction in pain with minimal systemic effects. In the infant population, in particular, local anesthetics provide a safe option for analgesia for pain.[56] For minor traumatic events (ie, lacerations requiring sutures), as well as major injuries requiring more painful intervention (ie, chest tubes insertion), local anesthesia can significantly reduce the perception of pain by blocking sodium-gated channels in nerve fibers.[57] Local anesthetics have few side effects and cause minimal hemodynamic perturbations in critically ill patients, which may make them ideal adjuvant therapies for the pediatric trauma patient. Of note, local anesthetics can produce cardiotoxic effects at higher doses. In a pediatric patient, the amount of local anesthetic is limited by the weight of the child to prevent effects on the cardiac sodium channels. Therefore, local anesthesia is not helpful for covering painful stimuli over large areas in children less than 10 kg due to volume limitation. PNBs, as well as central nerve blocks, are used with caution in pediatric trauma patients owing to concern for compartment syndrome.[58]

Acetaminophen is a safe and effective option for pain in the pediatric population. Although acetaminophen is not effective as a single agent for moderate to severe pain, it does have an opiate-sparing effect when administered as part of a balanced analgesic plan.[59] In 2010, the FDA approved IV acetaminophen for the treatment of pain and fever in pediatric patients. Although studies have failed to demonstrate superior pain control compared with oral acetaminophen in pediatric patients for pain, the IV formulation is useful in patients who are unable to take medications by mouth, such as trauma patients or patients who refuse oral medications. Pediatric patients treated with acetaminophen demonstrate decreased opioid utilization after surgery.[60]

NSAIDs (ie, ibuprofen, ketorolac, and naproxen) are an important component of pediatric trauma pain treatment. Due to inhibition of platelet function via COX-2, these agents are used cautiously in certain traumatic injuries. By decreasing release of prostaglandins and propagation of the inflammatory cascade, these medications provide a mechanism of action distinct from the other pain medications. Due to the inhibition of prostaglandins, which are required for osteogenesis, there has been concern about the effect of NSAIDs on posttrauma bone healing. In a comprehensive review of available studies examining the effect of NSAID usage on bone healing, there was no conclusive agreement of data supporting or refuting a negative impact on bone healing.[61] Thus, it is at the discretion of the clinician in weighing the benefits and risks for orthopedic traumatic injuries.

Ketamine is an NMDA-receptor antagonist that can decrease opioid usage in the management of moderate to severe pain.[62] Primate animal data demonstrates widespread apoptosis in the developing brain in subjects treated with ketamine.[63] However, other studies have demonstrated a decrease in pain-associated apoptosis, suggesting a protective effect of ketamine.[64] Ketamine also provides a sedative effect that relieves anxiety that can exacerbate pain symptoms in children.[65]

Another category of medication that can decrease the usage of opioids, are alpha-2 receptor agonists, such as clonidine and dexmedetomidine. This class of medication is also useful in prolonging the effects of neuraxial blocks and PNBs. Due to a reduction in catecholamine release and action on the locus ceruleus, these medications have sedative and anxiolytic properties without the risk of respiratory depression carried by opioids.

Benzodiazepines have a dual role in pediatric pain management. Not only can they help provide analgesia but they also have muscle relaxant and anxiolytic properties.[66] The various developmental stages of childhood may be associated with lacking or underdeveloped coping mechanisms.[67,68] In an uncontrolled and frightening situation, such as a traumatic injury, children experience significant stress and anxiety that may be misinterpreted as pain.[69] Benzodiazepines are useful in these situations because they not only provide analgesia but also alleviate anxiety, allowing for a more accurate assessment of pain. The muscle relaxant property occurs via gamma-aminobutyric acid (GABA) receptor agonism and this property may be beneficial in traumatic long bone injuries, particularly in the teenage patient with significant lean muscle tone.[67]

Opioids are a central medication in the treatment of severe pain for pediatric traumatic pain but should be used with caution owing to their potentially severe side effects. Infants exposed to morphine in the intensive care unit demonstrated decrease in brain growth, lower IQs, and impaired short-term memory on postdischarge follow-up visits. Some of these effects improve by 8 to 9 years of age but poor brain growth persists. Compounded by the current opioid abuse epidemic in the United States and that almost 5% of patients prescribed opioids will develop dependence, there should be a concerted effort to adequately treat pain using a multimodal and opioid-sparing approach.

SUMMARY

How do providers appropriately manage pain in the age of the opioid crisis? This question does not have a simple answer. It is imperative to find balance between achieving adequate pain control and minimizing opioid medications because the United States is experiencing devastating consequences resulting from the current opioid epidemic. Addressing psychosocial factors early on in a patient's trauma admission may improve long-term outcomes. The new focus of The Joint Commission is on frequently assessing pain and on not how well the patients subjectively feel their pain is being managed. Providing patients with education and expectations on pain control at time of admission may help in pain management during their hospitalization and postdischarge. It is important for patients to understand that a pain score of 0 in the initial postoperative or post-trauma period is unrealistic and that the goal of pain management is to sufficiently control pain so that they can comfortably and adequately participate in rehabilitative activities. It is crucial to recognize that there are different types of pain and various pathways through which they are mediated and that not all of them may respond to or require opioid analgesics. There should be an emphasis on using multimodal pain protocols that use regional techniques and medications (eg, gabapentin, acetaminophen, NSAIDs, and/or COX-2 inhibitors) to reduce the use of opioid medications and opioid prescriptions given on discharge. Finally, trauma centers should make efforts to develop standardized pain management protocols because they have been demonstrated to decrease the amount of opioids used in the outpatient setting while maintaining overall patient satisfaction and pain control.

REFERENCES

1. Campbell JN. Presidential address. Pain Forum 1996;5:85–8.
2. Joint Commission on Accreditation of Healthcare Organizations. Pain standards for 2001. CAMH Refreshed Core; 2001. Available at: https://jointcommission.org. Accessed April 24, 2018.

3. Joint Commission Resources. Comprehensive accreditation manual for hospitals. Oak Brook (IL): Joint Commission Resources; 2017.
4. The Joint Commission on Accreditation Survey. Available at: https://hcahpsonline. org. Accessed April 24, 2018.
5. Available at: https://www.qualitymeasures.ahrq.gov/summaries/summary/51203.
6. Yaster M, Benzon HT, Anderson TA. "Houston, we have a problem!": the role of the anesthesiologist in the current opioid epidemic. Anesth Analg 2017;125(5): 1429–31.
7. Cepeda MS, Africano JM, Polo R, et al. What decline in pain intensity is meaningful to patients with acute pain. Pain 2003;105:151–7.
8. Mathiesen O, Dahl B, Thomsen BA, et al. A comprehensive multimodal pain treatment reduces opioid consumption after multilevel spine surgery. Eur Spine J 2013;22:2089–96.
9. Volkow ND, McLellan AT. Opioid abuse in chronic pain-misconceptions and mitigation strategies. N Engl J Med 2016;374(13):1253–63.
10. Dworkin RH, O'Connor AB, Audette J, et al. Recommendations for the pharmacologic management of neuropathic pain: an overview and literature update. Mayo Clin Proc 2010;85(3 suppl):S3–14.
11. Tiippana EM, Hamunen K, Kontinen VK, et al. Do surgical patients benefit from perioperative gabapentin/pregabalin? A systematic review of efficacy and safety. Anesth Analg 2007;104(6):1545–56.
12. Woolf C. Pain: moving from symptom control toward mechanism-specific pharmacologic management. Ann Intern Med 2004;140:441–51.
13. National Vital Statistics System, Mortality. CDC wonder, Atlanta, GA: US Department of Health and Human Services, CDC; 2017. Available at: https://wonder. cdc.gov. Accessed April 24, 2018.
14. Florence CS, Zhou C, Luo F, et al. The economic burden of prescription opioid overdose, abuse, and dependence in the United States, 2013. Med Care 2016; 54(10):901–6.
15. Muhuri PK, Gfroerer JC, Davies MC. Associations of nonmedical pain reliever use and initiation of heroin use in the United States. CBHSQ Data Rev; 2013. Available at: http://samhsa.gov/data/. Accessed May, 2018.
16. Paulozzi L, Baldwin G, Franklin G, et al. CDC grand rounds: prescription drug overdoses—a US epidemic. MMWR Morb Mortal Wkly Rep 2012;61:10–3.
17. Paulozzi, et al. Vital signs: overdoses of prescriptions opioid pain relievers US 1999-2008. Morb Mortal Wkly Rep. Available at: www.cdc.gov. Accessed April 24, 2018.
18. Joint Commission Statement on Pain Management. 2016. Statement on pain management from David W. Baker, MD, MPH, FACP, Executive Vice President, healthcare quality evaluation, The Joint Commission. Available at: https://www. jointcommission.org. Accessed April 24, 2018.
19. Bricket MC, Long JJ, Pronovost PJ, et al. Prescription opioid analgesics commonly unused after surgery. JAMA Surg 2017;152(11):1066–71.
20. Cicero T, Inciardi J, Munoz A. Trends in abuse of OxyContin and other opioid analgesics in the United States: 2002–2004. J Pain 2005;6:662–72.
21. Webster L, Webster R. Predicting aberrant behaviors in opioid-treated patients. preliminary validation of the opioid risk tool. Pain Med 2005;6:432–42.
22. History of prescription drug monitoring programs. Available at: http://www. pdmpassist.org. Accessed March 30, 2018.
23. Reifler L, Droz D, Bailey JE, et al. Do prescription monitoring programs impact state trends in opioid abuse/misuse? Pain Med 2012;13:434–42.

24. Institute of Medicine. Relieving pain in America: a blueprint for transforming prevention, care, education, and research. Washington, DC: The National Academies Press; 2011. p. 129–30.

25. Chou R, Gordon DB, de Leon-Casasola OA, et al. Management of postoperative pain: a clinical practice guideline from the American Pain Society, the American Society of Regional Anesthesia and Pain Medicine, and the American Society of Anesthesiologists' Committee on Regional Anesthesia, Executive Committee, and Administrative Council. J Pain 2016;17(2):131–57.

26. Harford TC, Yi HY, Chen CM, et al. Substance use disorders and self- and other-directed violence among adults: results from the national survey on drug use and health. J Affect Disord 2018;225:365–73.

27. Cherpitel CJ, Ye Y, Andreuccetti G, et al. Risk of injury from alcohol, marijuana and other drug use among emergency department patients. Drug Alcohol Depend 2017;174:121–7.

28. Pain: current understanding of assessment, management, and treatments. American Pain Society; 2001. p. 1–91.

29. Gelfand HJ, Kent ML, Buckenmaier CC 3rd. Management of acute pain of the war wounded during short and long-distance transport and "Casevac". Tech Orthop 2017;32(4):263–9.

30. Todd KH. A review of current and emerging approaches to pain management in the emergency department. Pain Ther 2017;6(2):193–202.

31. Gros T, Viel E, Ripart J, et al. Prehospital analgesia with femoral nerve block following lower extremity injury. A 107 cases survey. Ann Fr Anesth Reanim 2012;31(11):846–9 [in French].

32. Dochez E, van Geffen GJ, Bruhn J, et al. Prehospital administered fascia iliaca compartment block by emergency medical service nurses, a feasibility study. Scand J Trauma Resusc Emerg Med 2014;22:38.

33. McRae PJ, Bendall JC, Madigan V, et al. Paramedic-performed fascia iliaca compartment block for femoral fractures: a controlled trial. J Emerg Med 2015; 48(5):581–9.

34. Simon BJ, Cushman J, Barraco R, et al. Pain management guidelines for blunt thoracic trauma. J Trauma 2005;59(5):1256–67.

35. McKendy KM, Lee LF, Boulva K, et al. Epidural analgesia for traumatic rib fractures is associated with worse outcomes: a matched analysis. J Surg Res 2017;214:117–23.

36. Galvagno SM Jr, Smith CE, Varon AJ, et al. Pain management for blunt thoracic trauma: a joint practice management guideline from the Eastern Association for the Surgery of Trauma and Trauma Anesthesiology Society. J Trauma Acute Care Surg 2016;81(5):936–51.

37. Kunhabdulla NP, Agarwal A, Gaur A, et al. Serratus anterior plane block for multiple rib fractures. Pain Physician 2014;17(4):E553–5.

38. Hamilton DL, Manickam B. Erector spinae plane block for pain relief in rib fractures. Br J Anaesth 2017;118(3):474–5.

39. Malekpour M, Hashmi A, Dove J, et al. Analgesic choice in management of rib fractures: paravertebral block or epidural analgesia? Anesth Analg 2017; 124(6):1906–11.

40. Nin OC, Patrick MR, Boezaart AP. The controversy of regional anesthesia, continuous peripheral nerve blocks, analgesia, and acute compartment syndrome. Tech Orthop 2017;32(4):243–7.

41. Mulroy MF, Daniel C. Moore, MD, the renaissance of regional anesthesia in North America. Reg Anesth Pain Med 2011;36(6):625–9.

42. Bonnet F, Marret RE. Effects of acetaminophen on morphine side effects and consumption after major surgery: meta analysis of randomized controlled trials. Br J Anaesth 2005;94:505–13.

43. Maund E, McDaid C, Rice S, et al. Paracetamol and selective and non-selective non-steroidal anti-inflammatory drugs for the reduction in morphine related side-effects after major surgery: a systematic review. Br J Anaesth 2011;106:292–7.

44. Gross J, et al. Reducing opioid use in trauma patients: a pain management protocol leads to fewer opioid prescriptions, better pain management, and greater patient satisfaction. Presented AAST Meeting. Baltimore, MD, September 15, 2018.

45. Hamilton BE, Hoyert DL, Martin JA, et al. Annual summary of vital statistics: 2010–2011. Pediatrics 2013;131(3):548–58.

46. American College of Surgeons Committee on Trauma. Advanced Trauma Life Support for Doctors (ATLS) student course manual. 8th edition. Chicago: American College of Surgeons; 2008. p. 225–45. Pediatric trauma.

47. Fitzgerald M. The development of nociceptive circuits. Nat Rev Neurosci 2005;6: 507–20.

48. Doesburg SM, Chau CM, Cheung TP, et al. Neonatal pain-related stress, functional cortical activity and visual-perceptual abilities in school-age children born at extremely low gestational age. Pain 2013;154(10):1946–52.

49. Yon JH, Daniel-Johnson J, Carter LB, et al. Anesthesia induces neuronal cell death in the developing rat brain via the intrinsic and extrinsic apoptotic pathways. Neuroscience 2005;135:815–27.

50. Taddio A, Shah V, Shah P, et al. Beta-endorphin concentration after administration of sucrose in preterm infants. Arch Pediatr Adolesc Med 2003;157:1071–4.

51. Malviya S, Polaner DM, Berde C. Acute pain. In: Cote CJ, Lerman J, Todres ID, editors. A practice of anesthesia for infants and children. Philadelphia: Saunders Elsevier; 2009. p. 939–78. OLD 47.

52. De Negri P, Ivani G, Tirri T, et al. New drugs, new techniques, new indications in pediatric regional anesthesia. Minerva Anestesiol 2002;68:420–7.

53. Harbaugh CM, Lee JS, Hu HM, et al. Persistent opioid use among pediatric patients after surgery. Pedatrics 2018;141(1):1–9.

54. Granry JC, Rod B, Monrigal JP, et al. The analgesic efficacy of an injectable prodrug of acetaminophen in children after orthopaedic surgery. Paediatr Anaesth 1997;7:445–9.

55. Lehr VT, Taddio A. Topical anesthesia in neonates: clinical practices and practical considerations. Semin Perinatol 2007;31:323–9.

56. Scholz A. Mechanisms of (local) anaesthetics on voltage-gated sodium and other ion channels. Br J Anaesth 2002;89(1):52–61.

57. Llewellyn N, Moriarty A. The national pediatric epidural audit. Paediatr Anaesth 2007;17:520–33.

58. Korpela R, Korvenoja P, Meretoja OA. Morphine-sparing effect of acetaminophen in pediatric day-case surgery. Anesthesiology 1999;91(2):442–7.

59. Ceelie I, de Wildt SN, van Dijk M. Effect of intravenous paracetamol on post-operative morphine requirements in neonates and infants undergoing major non-cardiac surgery. JAMA 2013;309(2):149–54.

60. Pountos I, Georgouli T, Calori GM, et al. Do nonsteroidal anti-inflammatory drugs affect bone healing? A critical analysis. ScientificWorldJournal 2012;2012: 606404.

61. Kaur S, Saroa R, Aggarwal S. Effect of intraoperative infusion of low-dose keta-mine on management of postoperative analgesia. J Nat Sci Biol Med 2015; 6(2):378–82.
62. Brambrink AM, Evers AS, Avidan MS, et al. Ketamine-induced neuroapoptosis in the fetal and neonatal rhesus macaque brain. Anesthesiology 2012;116:372–84.
63. Anand KJ, Garg S, Rovnaghi CR, et al. Ketamine reduces the cell death following inflammatory pain in newborn rat brain. Pediatr Res 2007;62:283–90.
64. Cho HK, Kim KW, Jeong YM, et al. Efficacy of ketamine in improving pain after tonsillectomy in children: meta-analysis. PLoS One 2014;9(6):e101259.
65. Migita R, Klein E, Garrison M. Sedation and analgesia for pediatric fracture reduction in the emergency department a systematic review. Arch Pediatr Ado-lesc Med 2006;160(1):46–51.
66. Joseph M, Brill J, Zeltzer L. Pediatric pain relief in trauma. Pediatr Rev 1999;20(3): 75–83.
67. Dahlquist LM, Gil KM, Armstrong D, et al. Preparing children for medical exam-inations: the importance of previous medical experience. Health Psychol 1986; 5:249–59.
68. Brophy CJ, Erickson MT. Children's self-statements and adjustment to elective outpatient surgery. J Dev Behav Pediatr 1990;11:13–6.
69. Zwicker JG, Miller SP, Grunau RE, et al. Morphine exposure is associated with altered cerebellar growth in premature newborns. Pediatric Academic Societies 2012;1528:465.

The Use of Point-of-Care Ultrasonography in Trauma Anesthesia

Davinder Ramsingh, MD[a],*, Venkat Reddy Mangunta, MD[b,c]

KEYWORDS

- Perioperative point-of-care ultrasound • Point-of-care ultrasonography in trauma
- Trauma anesthesia • Ultrasound education in anesthesia
- Ultrasound applications for trauma

KEY POINTS

- Management of the trauma patient requires rapid, coordinated care by anesthesiologists using various diagnostic or therapeutic modalities.
- Trauma anesthesiologists must become facile with the use of point-of-care ultrasound (POCUS) to maximize diagnosis and treatment of patients with traumatic injury.
- POCUS can assist in quickly diagnosing a multitude of traumatic injuries and differentiating diagnoses.
- Comprehensive POCUS educational curricula can assist anesthesiology residency programs in teaching residents this vital skillset.
- It is essential to the evolution of the specialty that anesthesiologists and anesthesiology training programs make POCUS education a priority.

INTRODUCTION

Caring for the trauma patient is one of the most complicated and high-risk patient care situations encountered by anesthesiologists. Around the world, trauma is the third leading cause of death overall, with more than 5 million deaths per year.[1] These

Disclosure Statement: Dr D. Ramsingh is a consultant for Edwards Life Sciences; Fujifilm Sonosite; and receives funds for research from General Electric on point-of-care ultrasound and anesthesia delivery systems, Merck Pharmaceuticals, Pacira Pharmaceuticals, Masimo Corporation, and Edwards Lifesciences. Dr V.R. Mangunta has no disclosures.

[a] Department of Anesthesiology, Loma Linda University School of Medicine, Loma Linda University Medical Center, 11234 Anderson Street, MC-2532-D, Loma Linda, CA 92354, USA; [b] Department of Anesthesiology, Division of Cardiovascular Anesthesia, Saint Luke's Mid America Heart Institute, University of Missouri-Kansas City School of Medicine, 4401 Wornall Road, Room 3103, Kansas City, MO 64111, USA; [c] Department of Anesthesiology, Division of Critical Care Medicine, Saint Luke's Mid America Heart Institute, University of Missouri-Kansas City School of Medicine, 4401 Wornall Road, Room 3103, Kansas City, MO 64111, USA
* Corresponding author.
E-mail address: DRamsingh@llu.edu

Anesthesiology Clin 37 (2019) 93–106
https://doi.org/10.1016/j.anclin.2018.09.011
1932-2275/19/© 2018 Elsevier Inc. All rights reserved.

anesthesiology.theclinics.com

patients often present in the middle of the night or on weekends when comprehensive resources and immediate consultation are not available. Therapy is often required for these patients for rapidly developing acute pathologic complications with little to no information on their past medical history. Furthermore, these patients may have rapid alterations to their cardiovascular and pulmonary status, and have a predisposition to occult injuries.

The management of the trauma patient requires rapid and coordinated care by trained physicians. Specialized training in trauma has undergone significant evolution over the past few decades. In 1990, Congress passed the Trauma Care Systems Planning and Development Act that led to the development of organized statewide trauma systems.[2] The American College of Surgeons (ACS) Committee on Trauma identified trauma centers as level I to level V, with the goal of ensuring that adequate resources and trauma-trained physicians are available to treat patients based on their severity of injury.[2] Additionally, the Advanced Trauma Life Support (ATLS) program has been adopted by the ACS and provides organized algorithms and approaches to managing trauma patients.[3]

Parallel to the development of highly reproducible algorithms for the treatment of trauma, ultrasound (US) technology has seen rapid evolution and expansion into emergency medicine (EM) training programs across the nation. EM physicians currently use bedside US for diagnostic and therapeutic purposes (eg, diagnosing hemothorax, retinal detachment). Point-of-care US (POCUS) has revolutionized the practice of emergency physicians.[4] The focused assessment with sonography for trauma (FAST)[5] examination has historically dominated the role of US in trauma management and remains the most studied example of focused clinical US.[6] However, over recent years, academic EM departments have greatly expanded the use of this technology from the periphery of trauma management to now include cardiopulmonary assessment, regional nerve blocks, and transesophageal echocardiography (TEE).

As much as EM has embraced this technology and developed focused applications for US use over the past decade, anesthesiology has lagged behind with regard to broadly adopting US technology. Although most anesthesiologists graduate residency with proficiency in performing US-guided regional anesthesia and vascular access, its use in the perioperative setting to quickly diagnose and aid in the treatment of emergent conditions (eg, pneumothorax, hemothorax, abdominal hemorrhage, hypovolemic or cardiogenic shock) has traditionally not been a focus of anesthesiology residency programs. By and large, anesthesia residents are graduating from residency with no formal education in the use of US for the acute diagnosis of adverse conditions in the perioperative setting.

The growing push for anesthesiologists to advance beyond their role in the intraoperative setting and realize their role as true perioperative physicians has led to the development of the subspecialty of trauma anesthesiology.[2] Since 2013, trauma anesthesiology has been recognized as a distinct subspecialty of anesthesiology by the American Society of Anesthesiologists (ASA).[2] In 2017, the ASA Committee on Trauma and Emergency Preparedness (COTEP) published the results of a survey demonstrating that there was significant disconnect between trauma surgeons and anesthesiologists regarding whether the anesthesiologists at their respective institutions were appropriately trained to manage trauma patients.[7] Trauma anesthesiologists must be prepared to emergently care for a patient with any severity of injury and must be adept at using the same management approaches described in the ATLS program. Development of POCUS curricula within anesthesiology residency programs is of paramount importance in the training of trauma anesthesiologists. This article reviews the topics of POCUS that are relevant to the perioperative trauma patient by reviewing the utility of POCUS for each category of the ATLS algorithm.

AIRWAY MANAGEMENT

The utility of POCUS for airway management has been demonstrated for the identification of difficult laryngoscopy, appropriate location of the endotracheal tube, and to facilitate cricothyrotomy or tracheostomy procedures.

Difficult Laryngoscopy and Endotracheal Tube Localization

POCUS has been demonstrated to improve the airway examination. Recently, Reddy and colleagues[8] found that anterior neck soft tissue thickness at the level of the vocal cords is a predictor of difficult airway. In addition to use of US for visualization of the hyoid bone, decreased temporomandibular joint mobility, measurement of the hyomental distance with neck extension, and the measurement of anterior soft tissue thickness at the thyrohyoid membrane have all been used to predict difficult airways.[9]

Endotracheal Tube Localization

US has demonstrated utility for verification of successful endotracheal intubation, reporting sensitivity and specificity of 100% versus esophageal intubation.[10] Because this is likely less of a concern in the perioperative setting, US has also demonstrated the ability to detect tracheal versus endobronchial intubation. Studies have demonstrated a higher degree of sensitivity and specificity (>93%) with POCUS than with auscultation.[11]

Cricothyrotomy or Tracheostomy

The use of surface landmarks to identify the cricothyroid membrane may be difficult, particularly for obese and female patients.[12,13] Bedside US is a reliable modality for rapid identification of anatomy for emergent cricothyrotomy.[14,15] Similarly, US has demonstrated improved success in accessing the trachea with more than 90% first-pass attempts.[16] The use of POCUS for percutaneous tracheostomies has demonstrated improved accuracy and has also been suggested to decrease complication rates.[17,18]

BREATHING OR PULMONARY

The ability of US to provide insight into pulmonary disease was previously thought to be impossible secondary to the acoustic impedance difference with aerated tissue. However, recent evidence has demonstrated POCUS to be extremely useful in establishing a differential diagnosis for acute respiratory failure in the postoperative period.[19] POCUS has proven to be faster and superior to chest radiograph (CXR) in diagnosing pneumothorax, pleural effusion, and alveolar interstitial diseases.[20,21] Ford and colleagues[22] recently demonstrated the ability of POCUS to detect perioperative pulmonary disease (atelectasis, consolidation, alveolar-interstitial syndrome, pleural effusion, and pneumothorax) in patients undergoing cardiac surgery with a high degree of specificity to CXR and physical examination findings. However, it is important to stress that a significant portion of pulmonary US deals with the detection and recognition of artifact generated by pathologic complications. This key point makes pulmonary US a challenging topic for the novice POCUS user.

Evaluation of Pneumothorax

US is highly accurate at detecting pneumothorax.[20,21] The primary US feature is the abolition of lung sliding, which is defined as the motion of visceral pleura against the parietal pleura during respiration. Importantly, this nonspecific finding is seen in several other conditions, such as malignancy, chronic obstructive pulmonary disease, and pneumonia. Additionally, it only detects pneumothoraces at the location at which the operator is scanning, thus it has the potential to miss pneumothoraces present at different scan locations. To this effect, it is important to scan the lung fields in more than one location. More specifically, it is the visualization of a lung point that is pathognomonic for pneumothorax. The lung point is the point at which the visceral pleura and parietal pleura separate. In a pneumothorax, both pleural layers separate. Tracing the pleural layer separation back to a lung point (point of separation) confirms that the lack of lung sliding is due to pneumothorax and not another disease process.

Parenchymal Lung Diseases

POCUS has demonstrated the same high degree of sensitivity for the detection of airspace disease within the lung parenchyma. Common practice in POCUS involves detecting artifacts generated from the disease developing within the lung parenchyma. Specifically, parenchyma diseases (edema, pneumonia, inflammation) will cause the interlobular septa to thicken, producing long vertical lines through the lung parenchyma on US imaging. This is commonly referred to as an US lung comet (ULC) (**Fig. 1**). Recent studies have demonstrated that the presence of greater than 9 ULCs per lung field is associated with 100% specificity for cardiogenic dyspnea.[23] Multiple protocols have been developed regarding pulmonary POCUS, mostly in the critical care setting. Of these, the bedside lung US in emergency (BLUE) protocol stands out as a comprehensive approach to rapidly facilitate the diagnosis of a patient in acute respiratory failure.[24]

Assessment for Pleural Effusion

US is more sensitive and specific than auscultation or CXR and is, therefore, the method of choice in detecting pleural effusion.[25,26] Effusions greater than 1 cm are easily detected and have a greater than 90% sensitivity and specificity for pleural effusion.[26] The utility for POCUS to guide thoracentesis has also been suggested.[27]

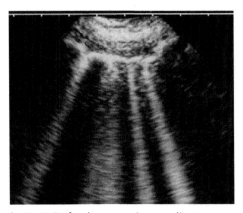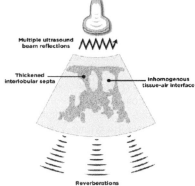

Fig. 1. ULC of pulmonary airspace disease.

CIRCULATION

POCUS has proven to be critical in the assessment of causes of hemodynamic instability and shock. Beyond assessing the patient's volume status, POCUS allows the anesthesiologist to differentiate between causes of shock and assess for injuries that may be leading to a shock state.

The following sections review the methods commonly used in POCUS that address these topics.

MECHANISMS OF HYPOTENSION

The FAST examination is the most widely used POCUS examination currently practiced in the acute care setting. This examination has been shown to very reliably detect greater than 200 mL of blood or fluid in body cavities (abdomen, pleural space, and pericardium) and it is a highly effective tool in the detection of clinically significant hemoperitoneum and hemopericardium in unstable patients.[5,28–30] Both trauma patients and patients in the postoperative care unit may have injuries that can cause significant blood loss and remain undetected by physical examination. The application of this examination allows the perioperative physician to determine if hemodynamic instability is secondary to pericardial and/or peritoneal injury, resulting in free fluid that can occur before or after surgery. Trauma patients can also sustain direct injury to their thoracic structures, such as the aorta or myocardium. A penetrating injury to the chest, for instance, may demonstrate an injury to the RV free wall, leading to a large pericardial effusion and tamponade. Additionally, elderly trauma patients with underlying ischemic heart disease are at risk for myocardial injury. POCUS can reveal new regional wall motion abnormalities in patients with previously normal cardiac function. In this way, obstructive (tamponade), hemorrhagic or hypovolemic, and cardiogenic causes of shock can quickly be elucidated by the perioperative physician.

Assessment of Cardiac Function

Transthoracic echocardiography (TTE) examination of the cardiopulmonary system using bedside POCUS technology has proven to be a reliable tool when compared with formal echocardiography.[31] Indeed, assessments of global left ventricular (LV) function, have shown a strong correlation ($r \geq 0.92$) between POCUS and formal echocardiography examinations.[31] Similarly, good correlation between POCUS and formal echocardiography was also shown when assessing right ventricular (RV) function and valvular function (excluding aortic stenosis) ($r > 0.81$).[31] Additional support for bedside TTE has been demonstrated in patients with shock in which adequate image quality was obtained in 99% of cases with a sensitivity and specificity approaching 100% and 95%, respectively, for identifying a cardiogenic cause for shock. Finally, it has been demonstrated that noncardiologists can be trained to perform and interpret a limited transthoracic examination focused on assessment of LV function.[32,33] Relatively straightforward measures of LV function can be obtained by obtaining parasternal short-axis views of the LV. By obtaining a parasternal short-axis view of the LV at the level of the papillary muscles, the operator can record a 2 to 4 beat video clip. The LV end-diastolic area (LVEDA) (**Fig. 2**A) and LV end-systolic area (LVESA) (**Fig. 2**B) can both be obtained by tracing the endocardial border using the trace function on the US. From this point, using the area measurements obtained, the fractional area change (FAC) can be calculated as follows:

FAC = [LVEDA – LVESA]/LVEDA.

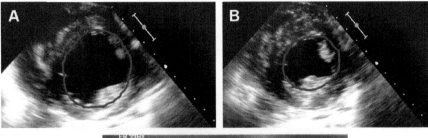

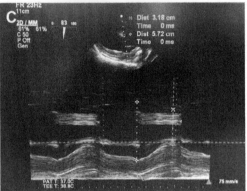

Fig. 2. Parasternal short-axis imaging. (*A, B*) Tracing of LVEDA and LVESA to calculate fractional area change and (*C*) M-mode to calculate fractional shortening. The red circle is a tracing of endocardial border in diastole (*A*) and systole (*B*). The green line is a tracing of the endocardial diameter in Motion Mode (*C*).

FAC is a two-dimensional assessment of LV function. A normal value ($\geq$50%) correlates to a normal LV ejection fraction ($\geq$55%). Alternatively, another basic measure of LV function, fractional shortening (FS), can also quickly be obtained from the same parasternal short-axis view, or the parasternal long-axis view just beyond the mitral valve at the level of the chordae tendineae. After this view is obtained, the Motion-mode beam is placed through the LV (**Fig. 2**C), taking care not to include the papillary muscles. Using the caliper tool on the US, the LV end-diastolic diameter (LVEDd) (5.72 cm in **Fig. 2**C) and LV end-systolic diameter (LVESd) (3.18 cm in **Fig. 2**C) are measured and the following equation is used:

FS = [LVEDd – LVESd]/LVEDd.

FS values greater than 30% are considered normal LV function. It is important to remember that both these measurements, FAC and FS, are affected by regional wall motion abnormalities. Additionally, FAC is essentially a 2-dimensional measurement and FS is a 1-dimensional measurement. Therefore, although they are useful insofar as providing a quick generalized assessment of LV systolic function, they do not provide a complete picture. The previous assessments are basic measures of systolic function and can be done by perioperative physicians with basic US training. Recently, guidelines have been published for cardiac POCUS by noncardiologists for the intensive care setting.[33] These guidelines can also be extended to the perioperative arena.

Volume Status

The concept of goal-directed fluid therapy is based on the evidence that either too little or too much fluid administration during the perioperative period can worsen a patient's clinical picture and/or organ function.[34] POCUS provides several techniques to assess static and dynamic indices of volume status. Regarding static indices, the diameter of the inferior vena cava (IVC) and its percent collapsibility from a maximal negative inspiratory breath has been shown to correlate to central venous pressures.[35,36] Another modality that can elucidate the volume status of a patient involves the direct measurement of LVEDA from a parasternal short-axis view (see **Fig. 2**A). Several studies have shown its utility in helping predict preload.[37–39]

Although these static parameters may be more reliable than urine output or other traditional identifiers of hypovolemia, they may not always predict fluid responsiveness. The Frank-Starling curve is an excellent depiction of the relationship between preload and cardiac output (**Fig. 3**). For increasing preload, cardiac output will increase to a point, after which no measurable increases in cardiac output will occur. Dynamic flow parameters are used to identify where on the Frank-Starling curve a patient exists. A patient on the steep portion (point A; see **Fig. 3**) of the Frank-Starling curve will respond to fluid by generating greater cardiac output (fluid-responsive). Alternatively, if the patient is on the flat portion of the curve (point B; see **Fig. 3**) there will be minimal increases in cardiac output for any further increases in preload. To assess a patient's location on the Frank-Starling curve and volume responsiveness, measurements must be made over several cardiac cycles. Patients subject to positive-pressure ventilation undergo regular changes in intrathoracic pressure that change loading conditions in the cardiovascular system. The greater the degree of intravascular volume depletion, the greater the effect positive-pressure ventilation has on RV (thereby LV) preload. Ideally, measurements are made before and after a volume challenge to assess for degree of response.

POCUS affords us several modalities to evaluate fluid responsiveness. Assessment of the IVC diameter change secondary to the mechanical ventilatory cycle has shown to predict fluid responsiveness. Specifically, the IVC diameter at end-expiration (D_{min}) and the IVC diameter at end-inspiration (D_{max}) can be measured to calculate the distensibility index of the IVC (dIVC) (**Fig. 4**A). Using a threshold dIVC of 18%, responders and nonresponders were discriminated with 90% sensitivity and 90% specificity in trauma patients presenting in shock.[40] More intricate dynamic methods of using POCUS to determine volume status include the use of Doppler ultrasonography (pulse-wave Doppler) to measure the stroke distance, which is termed velocity time

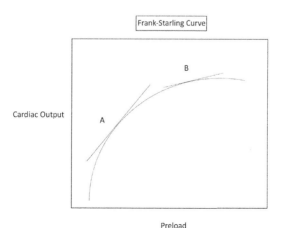

Fig. 3. Frank-Starling curve. Relationship between preload and cardiac output.

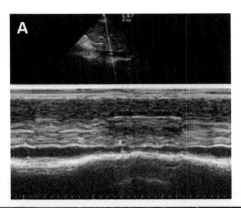

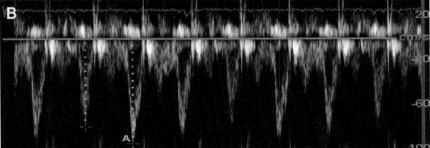

Fig. 4. US methods of volume status. (*A*) IVC collapsibility. (*B*) Doppler ultrasonography: velocity time integral variation.

integral (VTI), for the LV outflow tract (LVOT) or aorta. The stroke distance is essentially the measurement of the distance a volume of blood is moved, from point A to point B, with each ventricular contraction. By multiplying the stroke distance or VTI by the cross-sectional area of the tube through which the blood is flowing (LVOT in this example), the stroke volume (SV) is determined. Assuming no acute changes in LV contractility occur, the SV or LVOT VTIs can be compared during the inspiratory and expiratory phases of mechanical positive-pressure ventilation. A change in SV or VTI across LVOT during mechanical ventilation has been shown to indicate fluid responsiveness (**Fig. 4**B).[41,42] Likewise, the perioperative physician can ascertain where on the Frank-Starling curve their patient exists (volume-responsive steep segment or volume-nonresponsive flat segment) by measuring the SV or VTI before and after a fluid challenge. If a fluid challenge is given and the change in SV or VTI across the LVOT before and after is minimal, the patient is unlikely to respond to escalating amounts of fluid therapy.

DISABILITY OR NEUROLOGIC ASSESSMENT

There are many emerging areas in which POCUS can assist in the neurologic assessment of trauma patients. Probably among the most validated topics is using POCUS to estimate intracranial pressure (ICP) values. Visualizing the optic nerve sheath (ONS) and then measuring the ONS diameter has been shown to provide a rapid and accurate assessment of whether ICP is elevated. The ONS is contiguous with the dura mater and has a trabeculated arachnoid space through which cerebrospinal fluid circulates. The relationship between the ONS diameter (ONSD) and ICP has been well established.[43,44] The sensitivity for US in detecting elevated ICP was 100% (95% CI 68%–100%) and specificity was 63% (95% CI 50%–76%). An ONSD of greater than 5 mm, at a point approximately 2 mm from the retina, suggests elevated ICP. Additionally, rapid assessment of the retina and vitreous can reveal any obvious retinal detachment or vitreous hemorrhage that may have occurred due to trauma.

EXPOSURE OR ENVIRONMENT CONTROL
Gastric Content

The ability of POCUS to determine the volume of gastric content has emerged as a validated technique.[45] Perlas and colleagues[45] suggested that the presence of fluid in the gastric antrum identified on US in both the supine and right lateral decubitus positions may help identify patients at increased risk of aspiration. US can differentiate between solid and clear liquid stomach contents, with more particulate contents being associated with worsened outcomes if aspirated. Although healthy fasting patients may have gastric volumes of up to 1.5 mL/kg with minimal risk of aspiration, the visualization of gastric antrum fluid volumes of greater than 180 mL suggests patients may be at an increased risk for aspiration. The ability to detect gastric volume via POCUS may prove to be a valid method to aid in assessing aspiration risk, as well as determining if elective surgeries should be postponed based on the US examination findings.

Advanced Vascular Access

The use of US to assist with vascular access has advanced beyond its now widespread use for central venous access. Specifically, US has proven to reliably aid in the placement of difficult intravenous[46,47] and intraarterial catheters.[48,49] Use of US for peripheral venous access has also been shown to significantly increase success rates.[50] At the Mid America Heart Institute, US-guided access of the basilic vein and introduction of a guidewire followed by threading of a 4F vascular access sheath has reliably allowed preservation of the central veins for future access in patients with limited vascular access. A recent meta-analysis was conducted to compare US-guided and anatomic landmark-guided techniques for central venous catheter placement. The results demonstrated a decreased risk of cannulation failure, arterial puncture, hematoma, and hemothorax with the US-guided placement technique.[51]

In addition to US-guided vascular catheter placement, the Mid America Heart Institute's critical care and cardiovascular anesthesia providers use both POCUS and TEE to assist in the management of cardiac arrest and refractory acute respiratory distress syndrome (ARDS). TEE-guided insertion of a bicaval dual-lumen catheter into the right internal jugular vein by cardiac critical care anesthesiologists facilitates rapid transition to venovenous extracorporeal membrane oxygenation (ECMO) in severe ARDS. Similarly, during cardiac arrest and early cardiopulmonary resuscitation refractory to standard ACLS protocols, POCUS is used to guide the rapid placement of guidewires into the right femoral vein and left femoral artery for potential venoarterial ECMO cannulation by cardiothoracic surgeons in the operating room, if patients are candidates.

Evaluation of Deep Vein Thrombosis and Pulmonary Embolus

The current standard for evaluation of patients with suspected deep vein thrombosis or pulmonary embolus often involves lower compression ultrasonography and computed tomography pulmonary angiography. These tests are often performed despite low pretest probability and the long time to perform and obtain the results of these tests may contribute to diagnostic delays. Recent evidence supports that the use of a focused POCUS examination, performed by intensivists, involving lung US for subpleural infarcts, assessment for RV dilatation by cardiac US, and assessment for pulmonary embolus by leg vein US, can provide a high degree of sensitivity (90%) and specificity (86.2%) for the detection of pulmonary embolus.[52]

BRINGING THESE MODALITIES TO TRAUMA ANESTHESIOLOGISTS

Although it is encouraging to see the expansion of perioperative POCUS (P-POCUS), there remains the potential for tremendous growth with respect to the application of POCUS in trauma patient care. Other specialties have developed formalized educational and certification pathways.[53] EM has adopted POCUS training as a core competency for residency training and provides a year of fellowship training in clinical US. Of note, a similar interest in P-POCUS education has been reported by anesthesiology residents.[54]

Integration of comprehensive P-POCUS curricula has been developed for anesthesia residency training but is currently not widely adopted. The 2018 Accreditation Council for Graduate Medical Education program requirements for anesthesiology, however, now require "competency in using surface ultrasound and transesophageal and transthoracic echocardiography to guide the performance of invasive procedures and to evaluate organ function and pathology as related to anesthesia, critical care and resuscitation."[55] This change in educational requirements will encourage residency programs to adopt existing P-POCUS curricula. However, the effectiveness and efficacy of implementing P-POCUS into anesthesiology training program curricula remains to be determined. The implementation of POCUS training into anesthesiology residency programs still faces many obstacles, especially without standardized training protocols. It may take years for POCUS curricula to be effectively carried out and demonstrate proficient clinical skill levels and knowledge among trainees.

One study evaluated the utility of implementing a comprehensive POCUS educational curriculum for anesthesia residency training called Focused Perioperative Risk Evaluation Sonography Involving Gastro-Abdominal Hemodynamic and Transthoracic US (FORESIGHT). This curriculum incorporated the topics of

1. Cardiac
2. Pulmonary
3. Hemodynamic
4. Gastro-abdominal
5. Airway
6. Vascular access
7. ICP assessment

In this single-center study, implementation of the curriculum into residency training demonstrated statistical significance for positive participant satisfaction, improved knowledge, and acquisition of hands-on skills as evaluated via the Kirkpatrick assessment tool.[54] Additionally, a positive clinical impact was also suggested after 1 year of training. To further P-POCUS education, this curriculum is now online and provides open access, under a Creative Commons license (www.foresightultrasound.com).

This is among several initiatives to further the development of P-POCUS. Other initiatives include the focus-assessed TTE (FATE) protocol (http://usabcd.org), which was developed by an anesthesiologist and is among the most widely referenced POCUS examination protocols. Additional online resources available for education on P-POCUS include those from the Society of Critical Care Medicine (http://www.sccm.org/Education Center/Ultrasound/Pages/default.aspx), the American Institute of Ultrasound (http://www.aium.org), and various Continuing Medical Education training programs.[53]

Although these resources are important, the onus is on anesthesiologists to develop structured guidelines, endorsed educational pathways, and certified credentialing processes to incorporate P-POCUS into everyday practice. With the evolution of anesthesiology from a specialty relegated to the operative theater and intensive care units to a comprehensive perioperative role, anesthesiologists must embrace US technology and become leaders and educators in the development of new applications of this technology.

REFERENCES

1. American Association for the Surgery of Trauma; 2018. Available at: http://www.aast.org/trauma-facts. Accessed November 2, 2018.
2. Delegates ASoAHo. Statement of principles: trauma anesthesiology. American Society of Anesthesiologists House of Delegates; 2013. Available at: https://www.asahq.org/resources/resources-from-asa-committees/committee-on-trauma-and-emergency-preparedness/trauma-anesthesiology. Accessed November 2, 2018.
3. The Advanced Trauma Life Support. 2008. Available at: https://www.facs.org/quality-programs/trauma/atls.
4. Kendall JL, Hoffenberg SR, Smith RS. History of emergency and critical care ultrasound: the evolution of a new imaging paradigm. Crit Care Med 2007;35: S126–30.
5. Rozycki GS, Ochsner MG, Schmidt JA, et al. A prospective study of surgeon-performed ultrasound as the primary adjuvant modality for injured patient assessment. J Trauma 1995;39:492–8 [discussion: 498–500].
6. Gillman LM, Ball CG, Panebianco N, et al. Clinician performed resuscitative ultrasonography for the initial evaluation and resuscitation of trauma. Scand J Trauma Resusc Emerg Med 2009;17:34.
7. Kaslow O, Kuza CM, McCunn M, et al. Trauma anesthesiology as part of the core anesthesiology residency program training: expert opinion of the American Society of Anesthesiologists Committee on Trauma and emergency preparedness (ASA COTEP). Anesth Analg 2017;125:1060–5.
8. Reddy PB, Punetha P, Chalam KS. Ultrasonography - a viable tool for airway assessment. Indian J Anaesth 2016;60:807–13.
9. Fulkerson JS, Moore HM, Anderson TS, et al. Ultrasonography in the preoperative difficult airway assessment. J Clin Monit Comput 2017;31:513–30.
10. Muslu B, Sert H, Kaya A, et al. Use of sonography for rapid identification of esophageal and tracheal intubations in adult patients. J Ultrasound Med 2011; 30:671–6.
11. Ramsingh D, Frank E, Haughton E, et al. Auscultation versus point of care ultrasound to determine endotracheal versus bronchial intubation: a diagnostic accuracy study. Anesthesiology 2016;124(5):1012–20.
12. Elliott DS, Baker PA, Scott MR, et al. Accuracy of surface landmark identification for cannula cricothyroidotomy. Anaesthesia 2010;65:889–94.
13. Aslani A, Ng SC, Hurley M, et al. Accuracy of identification of the cricothyroid membrane in female subjects using palpation: an observational study. Anesth Analg 2012;114:987–92.

14. Nicholls SE, Sweeney TW, Ferre RM, et al. Bedside sonography by emergency physicians for the rapid identification of landmarks relevant to cricothyrotomy. Am J Emerg Med 2008;26:852–6.

15. Osman A, Sum KM. Role of upper airway ultrasound in airway management. J Intensive Care 2016;4:52.

16. Kleine-Brueggeney M, Greif R, Ross S, et al. Ultrasound-guided percutaneous tracheal puncture: a computer-tomographic controlled study in cadavers. Br J Anaesth 2011;106:738–42.

17. Rudas M, Seppelt I, Herkes R, et al. Traditional landmark versus ultrasound guided tracheal puncture during percutaneous dilatational tracheostomy in adult intensive care patients: a randomised controlled trial. Crit Care 2014;18:514.

18. Yavuz A, Yilmaz M, Goya C, et al. Advantages of US in percutaneous dilatational tracheostomy: randomized controlled trial and review of the literature. Radiology 2014;273:927–36.

19. Lee FC. Lung ultrasound-a primary survey of the acutely dyspneic patient. J Intensive Care 2016;4:57.

20. Xirouchaki N, Magkanas E, Vaporidi K, et al. Lung ultrasound in critically ill patients: comparison with bedside chest radiography. Intensive Care Med 2011; 37:1488–93.

21. Blaivas M, Lyon M, Duggal S. A prospective comparison of supine chest radiography and bedside ultrasound for the diagnosis of traumatic pneumothorax. Acad Emerg Med 2005;12:844–9.

22. Ford JW, Heiberg J, Brennan AP, et al. A pilot assessment of 3 point-of-care strategies for diagnosis of perioperative lung pathology. Anesth Analg 2017;124(3): 734–42.

23. Gargani L, Frassi F, Soldati G, et al. Ultrasound lung comets for the differential diagnosis of acute cardiogenic dyspnoea: a comparison with natriuretic peptides. Eur J Heart Fail 2008;10:70–7.

24. Lichtenstein DA, Meziere GA. Relevance of lung ultrasound in the diagnosis of acute respiratory failure: the BLUE protocol. Chest 2008;134:117–25.

25. Doust BD, Baum JK, Maklad NF, et al. Ultrasonic evaluation of pleural opacities. Radiology 1975;114:135–40.

26. Lichtenstein D, Goldstein I, Mourgeon E, et al. Comparative diagnostic performances of auscultation, chest radiography, and lung ultrasonography in acute respiratory distress syndrome. Anesthesiology 2004;100:9–15.

27. Lichtenstein D, Hulot JS, Rabiller A, et al. Feasibility and safety of ultrasound-aided thoracentesis in mechanically ventilated patients. Intensive Care Med 1999;25:955–8.

28. Scalea TM, Rodriguez A, Chiu WC, et al. Focused assessment with sonography for trauma (FAST): results from an international consensus conference. J Trauma 1999;46:466–72.

29. Rose JS. Ultrasound in abdominal trauma. Emerg Med Clin North Am 2004;22: 581–99, vii.

30. Kirkpatrick AW, Sirois M, Laupland KB, et al. Prospective evaluation of hand-held focused abdominal sonography for trauma (FAST) in blunt abdominal trauma. Can J Surg 2005;48:453–60.

31. Andersen GN, Haugen BO, Graven T, et al. Feasibility and reliability of point-of-care pocket-sized echocardiography. Eur J Echocardiogr 2011;12:665–70.

32. Manasia AR, Nagaraj HM, Kodali RB, et al. Feasibility and potential clinical utility of goal-directed transthoracic echocardiography performed by noncardiologist

intensivists using a small hand-carried device (SonoHeart) in critically ill patients. J Cardiothorac Vasc Anesth 2005;19:155–9.

33. Mazraeshahi RM, Farmer JC, Porembka DT. A suggested curriculum in echocardiography for critical care physicians. Crit Care Med 2007;35:S431–3.

34. Bundgaard-Nielsen M, Holte K, Secher NH, et al. Monitoring of peri-operative fluid administration by individualized goal-directed therapy. Acta Anaesthesiol Scand 2007;51:331–40.

35. Ommen SR, Nishimura RA, Hurrell DG, et al. Assessment of right atrial pressure with 2-dimensional and Doppler echocardiography: a simultaneous catheterization and echocardiographic study. Mayo Clin Proc 2000;75:24–9.

36. Prekker ME, Scott NL, Hart D, et al. Point-of-care ultrasound to estimate central venous pressure: a comparison of three techniques. Crit Care Med 2013;41: 833–41.

37. Cannesson M, Slieker J, Desebbe O, et al. Prediction of fluid responsiveness using respiratory variations in left ventricular stroke area by transoesophageal echocardiographic automated border detection in mechanically ventilated patients. Crit Care 2006;10:R171.

38. Scheuren K, Wente MN, Hainer C, et al. Left ventricular end-diastolic area is a measure of cardiac preload in patients with early septic shock. Eur J Anaesthesiol 2009;26:759–65.

39. Subramaniam B, Talmor D. Echocardiography for management of hypotension in the intensive care unit. Crit Care Med 2007;35:S401–7.

40. Sefidbakht S, Assadsangabi R, Abbasi HR, et al. Sonographic measurement of the inferior vena cava as a predictor of shock in trauma patients. Emerg Radiol 2007;14:181–5.

41. Broch O, Renner J, Gruenewald M, et al. Variation of left ventricular outflow tract velocity and global end-diastolic volume index reliably predict fluid responsiveness in cardiac surgery patients. J Crit Care 2012;27:325.e7-13.

42. Charron C, Caille V, Jardin F, et al. Echocardiographic measurement of fluid responsiveness. Curr Opin Crit Care 2006;12:249–54.

43. Hansen HC, Helmke K. Validation of the optic nerve sheath response to changing cerebrospinal fluid pressure: ultrasound findings during intrathecal infusion tests. J Neurosurg 1997;87:34–40.

44. Tayal VS, Neulander M, Norton HJ, et al. Emergency department sonographic measurement of optic nerve sheath diameter to detect findings of increased intracranial pressure in adult head injury patients. Ann Emerg Med 2007;49:508–14.

45. Perlas A, Van de Putte P, Van Houwe P, et al. I-AIM framework for point-of-care gastric ultrasound. Br J Anaesth 2016;116:7–11.

46. Costantino TG, Parikh AK, Satz WA, et al. Ultrasonography-guided peripheral intravenous access versus traditional approaches in patients with difficult intravenous access. Ann Emerg Med 2005;46:456–61.

47. Keyes LE, Frazee BW, Snoey ER, et al. Ultrasound-guided brachial and basilic vein cannulation in emergency department patients with difficult intravenous access. Ann Emerg Med 1999;34:711–4.

48. Ashworth A, Arrowsmith JE. Ultrasound-guided arterial cannulation. Eur J Anaesthesiol 2010;27:307.

49. Shiver S, Blaivas M, Lyon M. A prospective comparison of ultrasound-guided and blindly placed radial arterial catheters. Acad Emerg Med 2006;13:1275–9.

50. Stolz LA, Stolz U, Howe C, et al. Ultrasound-guided peripheral venous access: a meta-analysis and systematic review. J Vasc Access 2015;16(4):321–6.

51. Wu SY, Ling Q, Cao LH, et al. Real-time two-dimensional ultrasound guidance for central venous cannulation: a meta-analysis. Anesthesiology 2013;118:361–75.
52. Nazerian P, Vanni S, Volpicelli G, et al. Accuracy of point-of-care multiorgan ultrasonography for the diagnosis of pulmonary embolism. Chest 2014;145:950–7.
53. Mahmood F, Matyal R, Skubas N, et al. Perioperative ultrasound training in anesthesiology: a call to action. Anesth Analg 2016;122:1794–804.
54. Ramsingh D, Rinehart J, Kain Z, et al. Impact assessment of perioperative point-of-care ultrasound training on anesthesiology residents. Anesthesiology 2015; 123:670–82.
55. ACGME program requirements for graduate medical education in anesthesiology. Suite 2000, 401 North Michigan Avenue, Chicago, IL 60611. 2018. p. 17–8. Available at: https://www.acgme.org/Portals/0/PFAssets/ProgramRequirements/040Anesthesiology2018.pdf?ver=2018-06-14-142529-527. Accessed July 24, 2018.

Gender Disparities in Trauma Care

How Sex Determines Treatment, Behavior, and Outcome

Evie G. Marcolini, MD[a],*, Jennifer S. Albrecht, PhD[b],
Kinjal N. Sethuraman, MD, MPH[c], Lena M. Napolitano, MD, MCCM[d]

KEYWORDS

• Gender • Disparities • Trauma • Sex • Outcomes

KEY POINTS

• Sex differences in risk-taking behaviors have been associated with male sex, menstrual cycle timing, and cortisol levels.

• Differences in access to trauma services, including triage or transfer to a trauma center and level of medical attention, are associated with sex as well as race, rural versus urban location, and insurance status.

• Sex disparities have been shown to be associated with treatments such as venous thromboembolism prophylaxis and massive transfusion component ratios.

• US and European trauma database statistics as well as meta-analyses show sex differences associated with in-hospital mortality, multiple organ failure, pneumonia, and sepsis after trauma.

• National Trauma Databank and other literature show mixed results with respect to mortality after traumatic brain injury and its association with sex.

E.G. Marcolini and K.N. Sethuraman have no disclosures. Dr J.S. Albrecht was supported by Agency for Healthcare Research and Quality grant K01HS024560.
[a] Department of Surgery, Division of Emergency Medicine, University of Vermont College of Medicine, 111 Colchester Avenue, Burlington, VT 05401, USA; [b] Department of Epidemiology and Public Health, University of Maryland School of Medicine, MSTF 334C, 10. South Pine Street, Baltimore, MD 21201, USA; [c] Hyperbaric Medicine-Shock Trauma, University of Maryland, 22 South Greene Street, Baltimore, MD 21201, USA; [d] Acute Care Surgery [Trauma, Burn, Critical Care, Emergency Surgery], Department of Surgery, Trauma and Surgical Critical Care, University of Michigan Health System, University Hospital, Room 1C340, 1500 East Medical Center Drive, Ann Arbor, MI 48109-5033, USA
* Corresponding author.
E-mail address: emarcolini@gmail.com

Anesthesiology Clin 37 (2019) 107–117
https://doi.org/10.1016/j.anclin.2018.09.007
1932-2275/19/© 2018 Elsevier Inc. All rights reserved.

INTRODUCTION

The longstanding quest for improved outcome in trauma patients has supported research on the effect of sex on outcomes. Sex influences nearly everything from how we become trauma patients to how we are triaged, treated, and ultimately what our outcome will be. The term "sex" refers to biological characteristics and "gender" to social and cultural roles. Although these terms have different important meanings, they are mostly used interchangeably in the literature with little specific interrogation as to the different implications. Herein we use the term sex, and acknowledge that gender likely has important unexplored effects on trauma patients, or it may be buried within the existing data and is yet undifferentiated from sex.

The body of literature that examines these aspects is large. We present an overview of the findings with an eye to illuminating areas that are ripe for research. Trauma research is limited by the heterogeneity of its subject, but categorizing by sex may help move the field forward with improvement in outcomes.

We necessarily start from the beginning: what factors influence becoming a trauma patient? Does sex play a role? Next, do medical providers treat patients differently based on sex, and does that influence outcome? And, finally, we delve into the outcomes themselves and whether or not the literature can shed light on areas for improvement in both prevention and/or treatment.

RISK-TAKING BEHAVIOR

Sex differences in risk-taking behaviors have been well documented and studies continue to show that men and boys are more likely to have more severe injury than women and girls.[1–3] These differences have been attributed to increased testosterone levels in those with high risk tolerance.[4,5] Elevated testosterone levels are associated with decreased punishment sensitivity, showing a higher tolerance for consequences of risky behaviors.[6] Other studies have also suggested that risk aversion changes with phases of the menstrual cycle.[7] Studies outside of health and medicine also find similar changes to risk tolerance based on hormone levels. Sapienza and colleagues[8] showed that MBA students with higher salivary testosterone levels were more likely to have increased risk tolerance on a self-reported survey and take jobs that had a greater perceived element of risk in the job description.

The story of risk-taking behavior and hormones goes beyond testosterone alone. Changes in cortisol levels have also become a growing area of research with respect to sex and risk tolerance. Increases in stress-induced cortisol levels have been associated with increased risky behavior in men but not in women.[9,10] Weller and colleagues[11] demonstrated a change in risky behaviors in older healthy adults, based on an expected steep drop in cortisol levels throughout the day; if the drop in cortisol level was not as expected, the subject took more unnecessary risks.

A recent Canadian study by Asbridge and colleagues[12] showed adolescent boys who experience injury were more likely to smoke tobacco, drink alcohol, smoke marijuana, and have multiple sexual partners than girls who experience injury. In a 1999 meta-analysis of 150 articles, Byrnes[13] showed that men are more likely to engage in risky behaviors than women. Reudl and colleagues[14] showed that younger age and male sex were among the predictors of self-reported risk-taking behaviors in skiers and snowboarders. Men are also more likely to play competitive and recreational sports as adults compared with women, increasing exposure to potential injury.[15] Although there is a growing body of literature on distracted driving (cell phone use, texting, eating) the results for sex differences are mixed, with some self-reporting surveys indicating that women and younger subjects are more likely to report being distracted than men and older subjects (National Highway Safety Administration DOT HS 811 611),[16] but young men are more likely to engage in risky driving behavior. With advances in technology, focus on community-based education of new and younger drivers, and enforcement of distracted driving laws, crash rates may decrease regardless of sex.

The proclivity of men and boys to engage in risk-taking behaviors results in more severe injury. Unintentional overall nonfatal injury incidence between 2010 and 2016 was 8505 of 100,000 for female individuals and 10,176 of 100,000 for male individuals. The Centers for Disease Control and Prevention reported that in 2015, the age-adjusted mortality rate for men suffering violent injury was 30.6 of 100,000, whereas for women it was 9.2 of 100,000 (Web-based injury statistics query and reporting system: www.cdc.gov/injury/wisqars/index.html).

TRAUMA TREATMENT
Transfer to a Trauma Center

Sex disparities in access to services have been reported in many health care settings, including trauma care. A number of studies have documented that female sex is associated with decreased transfer rates from nontrauma centers (NTC) to trauma centers (TC). This is particularly concerning, as it has been clearly documented that initial triage to a TC leads to better overall outcomes.[17] A population-based analysis confirmed that initial triage of trauma patients to an NTC was associated with a 30% increase in mortality in the first 48 hours after injury.[18] When the differences in the provision of traumatic injury care start at the prehospital stage, current research would suggest that female patients may already be at a disadvantage for optimal long-term outcomes.

A population-based retrospective cohort analysis of severely injured adults showed that women receive less care from TCs than men.[19] Interestingly, the women in this study were older with more comorbidity, which would intuitively prompt most providers to seek higher levels of care. Emergency medical service personnel were less likely to transport female individuals from the field to a TC compared with male individuals. Similarly, physicians were less likely to transfer female patients to TCs compared with male patients, with adjusted odds of transfer to a TC that were 15% lower for female patients.

The reasons for this differential in access to trauma center care might be related to perceived difference in injury severity, likelihood of benefiting from trauma center care, or subconscious sex bias by health care personnel providing trauma care.

An interesting study of 15,906 patients with severe injury across 192 NTCs investigated the rate of transfer from NTC to TC based on the resource availability of the sending hospital (based on the availability of general and orthopedic surgeons, computed tomographic scanners, intensive care units, and emergency department staffing). Severely injured patients who received initial care in resource-rich NTCs were less likely to be transferred to a TC compared with resource-limited NTCs. The emergency department length of stay for trauma patients was also prolonged in resource-rich NTCs as compared with resource-limited NTCs.[20] Additional studies have documented a survival benefit among patients initially presenting to nontertiary (Level III or IV) TCs who are subsequently transferred to tertiary (Level I or II) TCs compared with those remaining in nontertiary TCs, even after adjusting for variables affecting the likelihood of transfer.[21] Because it has been documented that female patients are less likely than male patients to be transferred directly to TCs from the scene, it is of paramount importance to ensure appropriate transfer of female patients to TCs from NTCs when indicated.

In addition to sex, other factors have been identified that impact disparities in trauma care. African American, Hispanic, rural, and uninsured patients have worse outcomes after trauma, suggesting that these factors might modify the effect of sex on treatment and outcomes after trauma and result in even poorer outcomes for women with these characteristics.[22–24]

Treatment and Complications

Sex disparities in specific trauma treatments have also been identified. The proportion of trauma patients prescribed risk-appropriate venous thromboembolism (VTE) prophylaxis after trauma admission was significantly higher for male than female patients. After implementation of a mandatory clinical decision support system tool for VTE prophylaxis, disparities in best-practice VTE prophylaxis prescription were eliminated.[25]

In contrast to the previously mentioned study, use of high plasma:red blood cell (RBC) or platelet:RBC ratios in massive transfusion was associated with decreased 24-hour and 30-day mortality in male trauma patients, but there were no mortality differences noted in female patients. Although this difference may be related to sex-related differences in coagulability, further study is needed before implementing separate sex-specific protocols.[26]

TRAUMA OUTCOMES
General Trauma

In-hospital mortality

Studies examining the association between sex and mortality following trauma have been conducted primarily using trauma databases, which contain clinical and injury-related variables but do not provide information on death after discharge. Consequently, these studies have focused on in-hospital mortality and other in-hospital outcomes. Results have been mixed (**Table 1**). George and colleagues[27] conducted an analysis using data from the national trauma databank (NTDB) and reported that male sex was associated with increased odds of in-hospital mortality. In a related study, George and colleagues[28] performed a similar analysis focusing on an age-related sex differences in outcome and reported that among individuals younger than 50 years, male sex was associated with increased mortality. Haider and colleagues[29,30] performed 2 analyses using the NTDB to examine sex differences in mortality and complications following trauma. They reported that among adults hospitalized for ≥ 2 days there were decreased odds of mortality among women. When focusing on severely injured individuals with injury severity score (ISS) ≥ 16 and systolic blood pressure (SBP) <90 on admission, there were reduced odds of mortality among women.[29]

Liu and colleagues[31] reported that male sex was associated with increased mortality in a meta-analysis over 19 studies. Stratified analyses examining injury mechanism and severity, as well as age, did not significantly change estimates.

Trentzsch and colleagues[32] conducted 2 analyses of a large European trauma database to assess sex differences in in-hospital mortality and reported differing results. The first study showed that in 10,343 severely injured individuals, male sex was not associated with increased mortality. In a second study, Trentzsch and colleagues[33] matched men to women by age group, exact abbreviated injury scale (AIS) score for head, thorax, abdomen, and extremities, mechanism of injury, and prehospital presence of shock. Among the resulting 3887 matched pairs, male sex was associated with higher odds of mortality.[33] Napolitano and colleagues[34] showed that among patients aged 18 to 65, there were no sex differences in mortality when stratified by ISS score and age group. Sperry and colleagues[35] found no difference in adjusted mortality rates by sex in a secondary analysis of data from a multisite cohort study. Gannon and colleagues[36] reported that sex was not associated with mortality in a study of 22,332 individuals ages 18 to 65 years.

Table 1
Summary of studies on effect of sex on trauma mortality

Author	Study Design	Data Source	Sample	Injury	Findings
Gannon et al,[35] 2002	Retrospective cohort	All trauma centers in Pennsylvania, 1996–1997	N = 22,332, age 18–65	Blunt or penetrating trauma	No difference in mortality by sex
George et al,[26] 2003	Retrospective cohort	Single Level I trauma center, 1996–2001	N = 7438, age ≥16	Blunt or penetrating trauma	For those <50 with blunt injury, men had increased mortality (adjusted OR 2.5; 95% CI 1.3–4.9)
George et al,[27] 2003	Retrospective cohort	NTDB, 1994–1999	N = 175,702, age >19	Blunt or penetrating trauma	Men with blunt trauma had increased mortality (adjusted OR 1.49; 95% CI 1.39–1.59)
Sperry et al,[35] 2008	Retrospective cohort	Multisite cohort study, 2003–2007	N = 1036, age 16–90	Blunt, transfusion required	No difference in mortality by sex
Haider et al,[30] 2009	Retrospective cohort	NTDB, 2002–2006	N = 681,730, age ≥18	Hospital stay ≥3 d	Men had increased mortality (adjusted OR 1.27; 95% CI 1.20–1.32)
Haider et al,[29] 2010	Retrospective cohort	NTDB, 2001–2005	N = 43,010, age >12	Severe injury including ISS ≥16	Men aged 13–64 had increased mortality (adjusted OR 1.16; 95% CI 1.08–1.32). No difference ages >64
Trentzsch et al,[32] 2014	Retrospective cohort	German trauma registry, 2007–2012	N = 10,343, age ≥18	Blunt trauma, ISS ≥16, ≥3 d in ICU	No difference in mortality by sex
Trentzsch et al,[33] 2015	Retrospective cohort	German trauma registry, 1993–2006	N = 3887 matched male-female pairs, age ≥18	ISS ≥9	Men had increased mortality (OR 1.14; 95% CI 1.01–1.28); matching variables provided adjustment
Liu et al,[31] 2015	Meta-analysis	17 included studies with mortality outcomes		Blunt or penetrating trauma	Men had increased mortality (pooled RR 1.16; 95% CI 1.03–1.31)

Abbreviations: CI, confidence interval; ICU, intensive care unit; ISS, injury severity score; NTDB, national trauma databank; OR, odds ratio; RR, risk ratio.

Multiple organ failure

Multiple organ failure (MOF) following trauma was assessed in multiple studies that have consistently reported increased risk among men. Frohlich and colleagues[37] reported increased odds of MOF using data from a European trauma registry 2002 to 2011. Frink and colleagues[38] analyzed the association between sex and MOF using data from a Level I trauma center in Germany, 1997 to 2001, showing that male sex was associated with increased incidence of MOF in unadjusted analysis.

In addition to studies that focused specifically on MOF, many of the studies discussed previously examined outcomes in addition to mortality. In the 2 studies conducted by Trentzsch and colleagues, male sex was associated with increased odds of MOF.[12,32,33] In the analyses by Sperry and colleague[35] of severely injured trauma patients, women were at significantly decreased risk of MOF.[39] Finally, in the meta-analyses conducted by Liu and colleagues,[31] male sex was associated with increased risk of MOF.

Sepsis and pneumonia

Similar to results on MOF, results on pneumonia and sepsis have supported higher risk among male patients. Gannon and colleagues[40] showed that among patients aged 18 to 65 years, female sex was protective against pneumonia. In a prospective study conducted in 6 Level I TCs, male sex was independently associated with increased risk of ventilator-associated pneumonia.[41]

Two studies by Trentzsch and colleagues[32,33] documented increased risk of sepsis among men. Finally, the meta-analysis by Liu and colleagues[31] also reported increased risk of sepsis in men.

TRAUMATIC BRAIN INJURY

There continues to be significant research interest in sex differences in outcomes following traumatic brain injury (TBI).

Mortality at Hospital Discharge

Similar to results on sex differences in in-hospital mortality following trauma, results on sex differences in in-hospital mortality following TBI have been mixed. Berry and colleagues[42] used data from the NTDB 2000 to 2005, to assess sex differences in mortality among individuals with isolated moderate to severe TBI (defined as head AIS ≥3 and AIS for all other body parts <3), showing female sex to be associated with decreased odds of in-hospital mortality. The investigators also stratified by age to determine if menopausal status was associated with outcome. Compared with similarly aged men, women aged 45 to 54 years and those ≥55 years had reduced odds of mortality.[42] There was no sex difference in mortality among patients younger than 45 years. Davis and colleagues[43] reported similar results showing that women aged ≥50 years who were admitted to a trauma center for at least 24 hours had reduced risk of in-hospital mortality compared with men ≥50 years, whereas no sex difference in mortality was observed among adults younger than 50 years. In a study of elderly patients with TBI using the Nationwide Inpatient Sample, the highest mortality odds occurred in male patients.[44]

Leitgeb and colleagues[45] reported no sex differences in mortality among individuals with isolated moderate to severe TBI. Albrecht and colleagues[46] also reported no sex differences in mortality following isolated TBI among adults aged 65 and older using data from a trauma center 1996 to 2012. However, when the investigators included all patients with TBI, female sex was protective against in-hospital mortality.[46] The investigators concluded that severity of other injuries may have biased results from prior studies. In contrast with prior studies, Ottochian and colleagues[47] reported increased mortality among women with isolated severe TBI.

Long-Term Mortality

Harrison-Felix and colleagues[48] conducted 2 studies of long-term mortality among individuals with TBI who had received inpatient rehabilitation and had up to 12 years of follow-up. In one study using data from the TBI Model Systems National Database, sex was not significantly associated with long-term mortality. However, using data from a single hospital of individuals with TBI who had received inpatient rehabilitation and survived at least 1 year, male sex was associated with increased long-term mortality.[49]

Other Outcomes

Although much research effort has been devoted to better understanding sex differences in mortality following TBI, few studies have examined sex differences in other outcomes.

Neuropsychiatric disturbances such as depression and anxiety are common sequelae of TBI, but few studies have examined sex differences in risk of these outcomes.[50–53] In 2 studies using large administrative claims databases, Albrecht and colleagues[54,55] reported that although rates of depression were higher in women, TBI increased risk of depression in men more than in women. In related analyses that examined anxiety and posttraumatic stress disorder, Albrecht and colleagues[56] reported no sex differences in risk associated with TBI.

Sleep problems are also common following TBI, but few studies have examined sex differences in sleep disorders.[57,58] In a small study conducted by Mollayeva and colleagues[59] among patients with mild TBI, there were no sex differences in sleep disturbances. No sex differences in risk of ischemic stroke following TBI have been reported.[60–62] Similarly, no studies of dementia risk after TBI have reported incidence rates by sex or have evaluated sex as an effect modifier.[63–67]

SUMMARY

Results on sex differences in mortality following trauma are mixed, pointing to possible methodologic explanations. Men have different patterns of injury and higher severity, resulting in residual confounding of effect estimates despite best attempts to control for these factors. Furthermore, many studies control for factors that are in the causal pathway (eg, complications), introducing a possible source of bias. In contrast, evidence more consistently supports an association between male sex and increased risk of MOF, pneumonia, and sepsis. Investigation of the mechanisms of these differences will inform treatment efforts, including the possibility of sex-based treatment.

The inflammatory properties of sex hormones may contribute to trauma outcomes, but they do not fully explain observed sex differences.[41] High serum estradiol is a marker of injury severity and a predictor of death in the critically injured patient, regardless of sex. Whether or not estradiol plays a causal role in outcomes is unclear, but estrogen modulation represents a potential therapy for improving outcomes in critically ill trauma patients.[41,68]

Identification of sex disparities brings opportunities for improvement in many areas of health care, including trauma. Our research reveals significant areas of difference in treatment, behavior, and outcome for the trauma patient. We were not surprised by the results, but by the strength of the data. In spite of the inherent limitations of the data, some of the revelations may point toward areas for change in our systems and treatment, not in the least of which is the way that we as health care providers view our patients.

REFERENCES

1. Alexander CS, Somerfield MR, Ensminger ME, et al. Gender differences in injuries among rural youth. Inj Prev 1995;1(1):15–20.
2. Amarasingha N, Dissanayake S. Gender differences of young drivers on injury severity outcome of highway crashes. J Safety Res 2014;49:113–20.
3. Gescheit DT, Cormack SJ, Duffield R, et al. A multi-year injury epidemiology analysis of an elite national junior tennis program. J Sci Med Sport 2018. [Epub ahead of print].
4. Forbes EE, Dahl RE. Pubertal development and behavior: hormonal activation of social and motivational tendencies. Brain Cogn 2010;72(1):66–72.
5. Op de Macks ZA, Bunge SA, Bell ON, et al. Risky decision-making in adolescent girls: The role of pubertal hormones and reward circuitry. Psychoneuroendocrinology 2016;74:77–91.
6. Wu Y, Liu J, Qu L, et al. Single dose testosterone administration reduces loss chasing in healthy females. Psychoneuroendocrinology 2016;71:54–7.
7. Derntl B, Pintzinger N, Kryspin-Exner I, et al. The impact of sex hormone concentrations on decision-making in females and males. Front Neurosci 2014;8:352.
8. Sapienza P, Zingales L, Maestripieri D. Gender differences in financial risk aversion and career choices are affected by testosterone. Proc Natl Acad Sci U S A 2009;106(36):15268–73.
9. Kluen LM, Agorastos A, Wiedemann K, et al. Cortisol boosts risky decision-making behavior in men but not in women. Psychoneuroendocrinology 2017; 84:181–9.
10. van den Bos R, Taris R, Scheppink B, et al. Salivary cortisol and alpha-amylase levels during an assessment procedure correlate differently with risk-taking measures in male and female police recruits. Front Behav Neurosci 2013;7:219.
11. Weller JA, Buchanan TW, Shackleford C, et al. Diurnal cortisol rhythm is associated with increased risky decision-making in older adults. Psychol Aging 2014; 29(2):271–83.
12. Asbridge M, Azagba S, Langille DB, et al. Elevated depressive symptoms and adolescent injury: examining associations by injury frequency, injury type, and gender. BMC Public Health 2014;14:190.
13. Byrnes JP. Gender differences in risk taking: a meta-analysis. Psychol Bull 1999; 125(3):367–83.
14. Ruedl G, Burtscher M, Wolf M, et al. Are self-reported risk-taking behavior and helmet use associated with injury causes among skiers and snowboarders? Scand J Med Sci Sports 2015;25(1):125–30.
15. Deaner RO, Geary DC, Puts DA, et al. A sex difference in the predisposition for physical competition: males play sports much more than females even in the contemporary U.S. PLoS One 2012;7(11):e49168.
16. Available at: https://www.nhtsa.gov/sites/nhtsa.dot.gov/files/811611-youngdrivers report_highestlevel_phoneinvolvement.pdf.
17. MacKenzie EJ, Rivara FP, Jurkovich GJ, et al. A national evaluation of the effect of trauma-center care on mortality. N Engl J Med 2006;354(4):366–78.
18. Haas B, Stukel TA, Gomez D, et al. The mortality benefit of direct trauma center transport in a regional trauma system: a population-based analysis. J Trauma Acute Care Surg 2012;72(6):1510–5 [discussion: 1515–7].
19. Gomez D, Haas B, de Mestral C, et al. Gender-associated differences in access to trauma center care: a population-based analysis. Surgery 2012;152(2):179–85.

20. Gomez D, Haas B, de Mestral C, et al. Institutional and provider factors impeding access to trauma center care: an analysis of transfer practices in a regional trauma system. J Trauma acute Care Surg 2012;73(5):1288–93.

21. Garwe T, Cowan LD, Neas B, et al. Survival benefit of transfer to tertiary trauma centers for major trauma patients initially presenting to nontertiary trauma centers. Acad Emerg Med 2010;17(11):1223–32.

22. Haider AH, Chang DC, Efron DT, et al. Race and insurance status as risk factors for trauma mortality. Arch Surg 2008;143(10):945–9.

23. Hicks CW, Hashmi ZG, Hui X, et al. Explaining the paradoxical age-based racial disparities in survival after trauma: the role of the treating facility. Ann Surg 2015; 262(1):179–83.

24. Jarman MP, Castillo RC, Carlini AR, et al. Rural risk: geographic disparities in trauma mortality. Surgery 2016;160(6):1551–9.

25. Lau BD, Haider AH, Streiff MB, et al. Eliminating health care disparities with mandatory clinical decision support: the venous thromboembolism (VTE) example. Med Care 2015;53(1):18–24.

26. Rowell SE, Barbosa RR, Allison CE, et al. Gender-based differences in mortality in response to high product ratio massive transfusion. J Trauma 2011;71(2 Suppl 3): S375–9.

27. George RL, McGwin G Jr, Metzger J, et al. The association between gender and mortality among trauma patients as modified by age. J Trauma 2003;54(3): 464–71.

28. George RL, McGwin G Jr, Windham ST, et al. Age-related gender differential in outcome after blunt or penetrating trauma. Shock 2003;19(1):28–32.

29. Haider AH, Crompton JG, Chang DC, et al. Evidence of hormonal basis for improved survival among females with trauma-associated shock: an analysis of the National Trauma Data Bank. J Trauma 2010;69(3):537–40.

30. Haider AH, Crompton JG, Oyetunji T, et al. Females have fewer complications and lower mortality following trauma than similarly injured males: a risk adjusted analysis of adults in the National Trauma Data Bank. Surgery 2009;146(2): 308–15.

31. Liu T, Xie J, Yang F, et al. The influence of sex on outcomes in trauma patients: a meta-analysis. Am J Surg 2015;210(5):911–21.

32. Trentzsch H, Nienaber U, Behnke M, et al. Female sex protects from organ failure and sepsis after major trauma haemorrhage. Injury 2014;45(Suppl 3):S20–8.

33. Trentzsch H, Lefering R, Nienaber U, et al. The role of biological sex in severely traumatized patients on outcomes: a matched-pair analysis. Ann Surg 2015; 261(4):774–80.

34. Napolitano LM, Greco ME, Rodriguez A, et al. Gender differences in adverse outcomes after blunt trauma. J Trauma 2001;50(2):274–80.

35. Sperry JL, Nathens AB, Frankel HL, et al. Characterization of the gender dimorphism after injury and hemorrhagic shock: are hormonal differences responsible? Crit Care Med 2008;36(6):1838–45.

36. Gannon CJ, Napolitano LM, Pasquale M, et al. A statewide population-based study of gender differences in trauma: validation of a prior single-institution study J Am Coll Surg 2002;195(1):11–8.

37. Frohlich M, Lefering R, Probst C, et al. Epidemiology and risk factors of multiple-organ failure after multiple trauma: an analysis of 31,154 patients from the TraumaRegister DGU. J Trauma Acute Care Surg 2014;76(4):921–7 [discussion: 927–8].

38. Frink M, Pape HC, van Griensven M, et al. Influence of sex and age on mods and cytokines after multiple injuries. Shock 2007;27(2):151–6.

39. Marshall JC, Cook DJ, Christou NV, et al. Multiple organ dysfunction score: a reliable descriptor of a complex clinical outcome. Crit Care Med 1995;23(10): 1638–52.

40. Gannon CJ, Pasquale M, Tracy JK, et al. Male gender is associated with increased risk for postinjury pneumonia. Shock 2004;21(5):410–4.

41. Croce MA, Brasel KJ, Coimbra R, et al. National Trauma Institute prospective evaluation of the ventilator bundle in trauma patients: does it really work? J Trauma Acute Care Surg 2013;74(2):354–60 [discussion: 360–52].

42. Berry C, Ley EJ, Tillou A, et al. The effect of gender on patients with moderate to severe head injuries. J Trauma 2009;67(5):950–3.

43. Davis DP, Douglas DJ, Smith W, et al. Traumatic brain injury outcomes in pre- and post- menopausal females versus age-matched males. J Neurotrauma 2006; 23(2):140–8.

44. Haring RS, Narang K, Canner JK, et al. Traumatic brain injury in the elderly: morbidity and mortality trends and risk factors. J Surg Res 2015;195(1):1–9.

45. Leitgeb J, Mauritz W, Brazinova A, et al. Effects of gender on outcomes after traumatic brain injury. J Trauma 2011;71(6):1620–6.

46. Albrecht JS, McCunn M, Stein DM, et al. Sex differences in mortality following isolated traumatic brain injury among older adults. J Trauma Acute Care Surg 2016; 81(3):486–92.

47. Ottochian M, Salim A, Berry C, et al. Severe traumatic brain injury: is there a gender difference in mortality? Am J Surg 2009;197(2):155–8.

48. Harrison-Felix C, Whiteneck G, DeVivo M, et al. Mortality following rehabilitation in the traumatic brain injury model systems of care. NeuroRehabilitation 2004;19(1): 45–54.

49. Harrison-Felix CL, Whiteneck GG, Jha A, et al. Mortality over four decades after traumatic brain injury rehabilitation: a retrospective cohort study. Arch Phys Med Rehabil 2009;90(9):1506–13.

50. Bryant RA, O'Donnell ML, Creamer M, et al. The psychiatric sequelae of traumatic injury. Am J Psychiatry 2010;167(3):312–20.

51. Deb S, Lyons I, Koutzoukis C, et al. Rate of psychiatric illness 1 year after traumatic brain injury. Am J Psychiatry 1999;156(3):374–8.

52. Jorge RE, Robinson RG, Moser D, et al. Major depression following traumatic brain injury. Arch Gen Psychiatry 2004;61(1):42–50.

53. Rapoport MJ. Depression following traumatic brain injury: epidemiology, risk factors and management. CNS Drugs 2012;26(2):111–21.

54. Albrecht JS, Barbour L, Abariga SA, et al. Risk of depression following traumatic brain injury in a large national sample. J Neurotrauma 2018. [Epub ahead of print].

55. Albrecht JS, Kiptanui Z, Tsang Y, et al. Depression among older adults after traumatic brain injury: a national analysis. Am J Geriatr Psychiatry 2015;23(6): 607–14.

56. Albrecht JS, Peters ME, Smith GS, et al. Anxiety and posttraumatic stress disorder among medicare beneficiaries after traumatic brain injury. J Head Trauma Rehabil 2017;32(3):178–84.

57. Wickwire E, Schnyer DM, Germain A, et al. Sleep, sleep disorders, and circadian health following mild traumatic brain injury: review and research agenda. J Neurotrauma 2018. [Epub ahead of print].

58. Wickwire EM, Williams SG, Roth T, et al. Sleep, sleep disorders, and mild traumatic brain injury. What we know and what we need to know: findings from a national working group. Neurotherapeutics 2016;13(2):403–17.

59. Mollayeva T, Colantonio A, Cassidy JD, et al. Sleep stage distribution in persons with mild traumatic brain injury: a polysomnographic study according to American Academy of Sleep Medicine standards. Sleep Med 2017;34:179–92.

60. Albrecht JS, Liu X, Smith GS, et al. Stroke incidence following traumatic brain injury in older adults. J Head Trauma Rehabil 2015;30(2):E62–7.

61. Burke JF, Stulc JL, Skolarus LE, et al. Traumatic brain injury may be an independent risk factor for stroke. Neurology 2013;81(1):33–9.

62. Chen YH, Kang JH, Lin HC. Patients with traumatic brain injury: population-based study suggests increased risk of stroke. Stroke 2011;42(10):2733–9.

63. Barnes DE, Byers AL, Gardner RC, et al. Association of mild traumatic brain injury with and without loss of consciousness with dementia in US military veterans. JAMA Neurol 2018;75(9):1055–61.

64. Barnes DE, Kaup A, Kirby KA, et al. Traumatic brain injury and risk of dementia in older veterans. Neurology 2014;83(4):312–9.

65. Dams-O'Connor K, Gibbons LE, Bowen JD, et al. Risk for late-life re-injury, dementia and death among individuals with traumatic brain injury: a population-based study. J Neurol Neurosurg Psychiatry 2013;84(2):177–82.

66. Gardner RC, Burke JF, Nettiksimmons J, et al. Dementia risk after traumatic brain injury vs nonbrain trauma: the role of age and severity. JAMA Neurol 2014;71(12):1490–7.

67. Plassman BL, Havlik RJ, Steffens DC, et al. Documented head injury in early adulthood and risk of Alzheimer's disease and other dementias. Neurology 2000;55(8):1158–66.

68. Heffernan DS, Dossett LA, Lightfoot MA, et al. Gender and acute respiratory distress syndrome in critically injured adults: a prospective study. J Trauma 2011;71(4):878–83 [discussion: 883–75].

Pediatric Traumatic Brain Injury and Associated Topics

An Overview of Abusive Head Trauma, Nonaccidental Trauma, and Sports Concussions

Erik B. Smith, MD, JD, MS[a],*, Jennifer K. Lee, MD[a],
Monica S. Vavilala, MD[b], Sarah A. Lee, MD[b]

KEYWORDS

- Child abuse • Brain injuries • Sports-related head injury • Mild traumatic brain injury
- Concussion • Preoperative evaluation • SCAT-3

KEY POINTS

- Nonaccidental trauma must be considered in all pediatric trauma cases.
- Abusive head trauma is the most common cause of death from child abuse.
- Perioperative and intensive care unit management of pediatric traumatic brain injury (TBI) aims to ensure adequate cerebral perfusion, prevention of hypoxia and hypercarbia, and aggressive control of intracranial pressure and core temperature.
- Children with sports-related TBI who undergo surgery and anesthesia soon after injury may be vulnerable to worsening neurologic injury caused by impaired cerebral autoregulation, among other effects.
- It is important to screen for potential TBI in sports-related injuries and factor in perioperative management.

NONACCIDENTAL TRAUMA AND ABUSIVE HEAD TRAUMA

Nonaccidental trauma (NAT) is a leading cause of preventable death in the pediatric population. Abusive head trauma (AHT) is the most common cause of NAT related mortality. Clinicians must always consider abuse in their differential diagnosis when

Disclosures: J.K. Lee received research support from Medtronic and was also a paid advisory board member for Medtronic. This arrangement has been reviewed and approved by the Johns Hopkins University in accordance with its conflict of interest policies. All other authors have no disclosures.
[a] Department of Anesthesiology and Critical Care Medicine, Division of Pediatric Anesthesiology, Johns Hopkins University, 1800 Orleans Street, Baltimore, MD 21287, USA; [b] Department of Anesthesiology, University of Washington, Harborview Medical Center, 325 Ninth Avenue, Seattle, WA 98104, USA
* Corresponding author.
E-mail address: erik@jhmi.edu

evaluating and treating children, particularly when the mechanism of injury is unclear or when reported history does not match the injuries or the child's developmental age.

Definitions

Child abuse, child neglect, child maltreatment, and NAT are often used interchangeably. Although subtle distinctions apply, the authors recommend use of the inclusive "child abuse and neglect" definition by the US Centers for Disease Control and Prevention: "Any act or series of acts of commission or omission by a parent or other caregiver that results in harm, potential for harm, or threat of harm to a child."[1,2] NAT is the commission subset of this definition. AHT is a subset of NAT. The American Academy of Pediatrics defines AHT as "the constellation of cerebral, spinal, and cranial injuries that result from inflicted head injury to infants and young children."[3]

Epidemiology of Nonaccidental Trauma and Abusive Head Trauma

In 2016 the US Department of Health and Human Services (HHS) estimated a yearly death rate from child abuse of 2.36 per 100,000 children. Children younger than one year old are at highest risk of death, with a ten-fold greater rate of abuse-related mortality compared with older children.[4] Because of the difficulty of identifying abuse cases and variation in data collection, these are likely underestimates.[5] AHT is not directly tracked by HHS despite AHT being the deadliest form of child abuse and the most common cause of severe traumatic brain injury (TBI) in infants.[6] One nongovernmental study estimated the yearly rate of AHT at 27.5 to 32.2 per 100,000 infants less than one year old.[7] Children between two and seven years old can also suffer from AHT, albeit it at a lower rate than that of infants.[8]

Legal Reporting Recommendations and Requirements

All US states have statutes requiring clinicians to report suspected or known child abuse. The criteria, standards, and circumstances vary by state. Some states have criminal penalties for failing to report child abuse. Clinicians reporting suspected abuse are immune from criminal and civil liability pursuant to the federal Child Abuse Prevention and Treatment Act of 1974.[9]

Nonaccidental Trauma Injury Overview

NAT includes trauma to the head, abdomen, mouth, esophagus, sex organs, bones, and skin. Sexual abuse can be a contributing factor. Minor abuse may precede major abuse. Sentinel abuse signs may foreshadow a future catastrophe; therefore, recognizing a sentinel sign and taking action can save a child's life and rescue other at-risk children in the household. One study showed that sentinel signs of injury were present in 30% of infants with AHT (**Table 1**).

Table 1 Sentinel injuries observed in infants with abusive head trauma, with incidence on presentation	
Bruising (face, forehead, ear, extremity, trunk)	80%
Intraoral injury (frenulum injury, tongue contusion)	11%
Fracture (including both acute and healing)	7%

Data from Sheets LK, Leach ME, Koszewski IJ, et al. Sentinel injuries in infants evaluated for child physical abuse. Pediatrics 2013;131(4):701–7.

Nonaccidental Trauma Management, Examination, Documentation, and Referral

Management starts with constant awareness and vigilance for signs of potential abuse. Identifying NAT and AHT are not core competencies in anesthesia education, and education about abuse must be improved. Anesthesiologists often care for infants and children soon after traumatic injury during the critical time frame when signs of recent or chronic abuse are still visible. Clinicians should conduct thorough head-to-toe skin examinations during patient undressing for surgery (**Box 1**).

Routine clinical care may alter physical evidence of abuse and can confound investigation. Such care interventions include line placement, intubation, Foley catheter placement, skin preparation, surgery, and bandaging. Anesthesiologists and operating room teams must document evidence of abuse before beginning clinical procedures (**Table 2**).

Child abuse pediatricians work with interdisciplinary teams that include social workers and the police. They can guide forensic examination, advise on documentation and collection of evidence, and provide work-up continuity.

Box 1
Skin lesions associated with abuse

Bruises in early and late stages of healing

Patterns: loops, belts or belt buckles, cords, cigarette burns, hand prints, finger prints

Tongue and lip injuries: may be from forcing a utensil or object into the child's mouth

Lacerations in different stages of healing

Bruises in a child who cannot walk or who has limited mobility

Data from Ward MG, Ornstein A, Niec A, et al. The medical assessment of bruising in suspected child maltreatment cases: A clinical perspective. Paediatr Child Health 2013;18(8):433–42.

Table 2
Documentation before initiating clinical care that could alter skin findings

Take photographs of skin lesions	• Use HIPAA-compliant methods • Place rulers or an object of consistent size (eg, a coin) next to the lesion in the photograph • Label the photograph with key information. For example, write "right lower leg" on a piece of paper in the photograph
Describe skin lesions with location and size	• Draw a body outline and note lesion locations • Estimate the lesion's size (eg, the size of a quarter) • Record colors and other characteristics of the lesion • Scan this drawing into the medical record
Document genital and perianal injuries	• Signs of sexual abuse may be distorted by Foley catheter placement • Burns from dipping/immersion may be on the perineum (and bottom of feet)
Use plain language that people without medical knowledge can understand	• Eg, use the word "bruise" instead of "hematoma," and "bleeding" rather than "hemorrhage" • This information may be used during the investigation and in court
Report concerns of abuse	• Ensure the surgeons, hospitalists, and the child's pediatrician are aware of the documentation and concerns • Contact the institutional child protection team, or notify the appropriate authorities • Inform investigators where the relevant information is located in the medical chart

Abbreviation: HIPAA, Health Insurance Portability and Accountability Act.

Skin Injuries

Skin injuries, such as bruises, are the most common manifestation of child abuse and the most common sentinel injury.[10,11] Bruises can also occur from normal pediatric behavior, and bleeding disorders can make bruising more severe. Bruise-like skin findings may also be congenital malformations, dyes and inks, or side effects of cultural practices such as cupping.[11]

Babies less than nine months old are younger than cruising age and rarely show bruising (1% compared with 40% to 90% of children older than nine months old). Most accidental bruises are small, oval, and associated with a bony prominence. Abusive bruises are associated with patterned imprints of inflicting objects, such as hands, fingers, belts, and shoe soles. Bruises in various stages of healing are also associated with abuse (**Box 1**).[11]

Abusive Trauma of the Abdomen, Oral Cavity, and Esophagus

More than half of child abuse cases involve trauma to the head, face, or neck. Intraoral injuries account for 12% of documented abuse injuries; however, this likely underestimates the true rate because of poor clinician awareness of how to assess intraoral injuries and the frequent absence of additional abuse signs. Concerning signs include dental neglect, dental trauma, mucosal injuries, tongue lacerations, and frenulum injury.[5] Intraoral injuries may be associated with sexual abuse.

Abdominal trauma may include splenic injury, liver lacerations, or duodenal injury that present as bowel obstruction, hematoma, or stricture. Note that one-third of pediatric abdominal injuries from abuse do not have visible external signs of injury.[12]

Abusive Orthopedic Injuries

Orthopedic injuries can involve any bones, including the skull, spine, ribs, and long bones.[13] A radiographic full-body skeletal survey is critical when evaluating suspected abuse, especially in children younger than two years old.[13] Skeletal surveys may reveal subtle abuse injuries, including fracture fragments at the growth plate, growth plate irregularities, and subperiosteal new bone formation.[14]

Abusive Head Trauma

AHT is the deadliest form of nonaccidental trauma. It can happen to any child in any family or care setting. Some studies suggest increased AHT risk with young parents, delays in prenatal care, low birth weight, and socioeconomic stress.[15,16] The AHT perpetrator is often but not always a parent. **Box 2** lists confessions that describe acts of AHT.

Box 2
Confessions from perpetrators of abusive head trauma

I didn't want to choke him, but I wanted him to stop crying. I picked him up and I shook him; I threw him on the bed and he bounced on the sheet.

I shook her so she'd be quiet, it lasted maybe 5 minutes; I was exasperated; I shook her up and down, in front of me, without holding her against me; I was shaking her hard; I was crying just like she was, and I was worked up.

Data from Adamsbaum C, Grabar S, Mejean N, et al. Abusive head trauma: judicial admissions highlight violent and repetitive shaking. Pediatrics 2010;126(3):546–55.

Diagnosis and Recognition of Abusive Head Trauma

AHT is missed in one-third of cases despite signs of head trauma, including vomiting, irritability, superficial face and scalp injuries, seizures, or respiratory abnormalities.[17] Misdiagnoses attributed these findings to a medical process or accidental injury.[17] Socioeconomic cognitive bias may play a role. Of missed AHT cases, families tend to be younger, white, and have two parents living with the child.[17]

Families or guardians accompanying the victim may present vague stories that are inconsistent with the observed injury. One AHT study that analyzed perpetrator confessions found that cases involved a single shaking episode in 45% of cases and repeated episodes in 55%, with a range of two to 30 episodes. In some cases, shaking was habitual for weeks or months and was often in response to the baby crying. Perpetrators often said the child would sleep after shaking, which led to habitual repeated shaking episodes. Some described verbal abuse and others described blunt impact to the head. Almost all cases involved a significant delay between the abuse and bringing the child to medical care.[18]

Clinical findings associated with AHT include subdural hematoma, hypoxic ischemic encephalopathy, and bilateral retinal hemorrhage (**Figs. 1–3**). The mechanisms and presentation AHT are complex (**Table 3**). Altered mental status may manifest as irritability, inconsolable crying, or drowsiness. Rapid brain degeneration with multifocal leukoencephalopathy and diffuse atrophy has been described

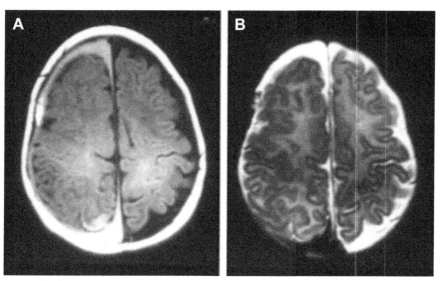

Fig. 1. Abusive head trauma. Axial T1-weighted (*A*) and T2-weighted (*B*) MRI scans of an infant reveal bilateral subdural blood collections of different ages. Right collection shows blood in the late subacute phase (2–4 weeks old), and left shows blood in the chronic phase (>1 month). This finding is highly suggestive of repeated abuse. (*From* Michelson DJ, Ashwal S. Neuroimaging. In: Vincent JL, Abraham E, Moore FA, et al, editors. Textbook of critical care. 6th edition. Philadelphia: Saunders; 2011; with permission.)

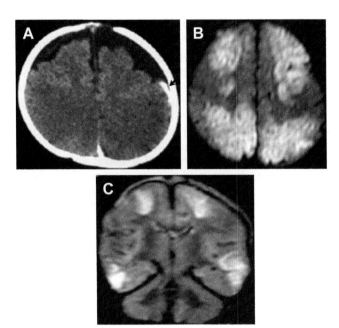

Fig. 2. Watershed pattern of supratentorial hypoxic ischemic injury. Four-month-old boy with acute mental status change and seizures. (*A*) Computed tomography on admission to the emergency room shows bilateral chronic subdural collections with evidence of acute bleed on the left (*arrow*). Loss of gray-white matter discrimination because of cortical edema is present bilaterally. (*B*) MRI axial diffusion, B1000, shows bilateral watershed areas of restricted diffusion in watershed distribution. (*C*) MRI coronal diffusion, B1000, shows bilateral watershed areas of restricted diffusion. (*From* Zimmerman RA, Bilaniuk LT, Farina L. Non-accidental brain trauma in infants: diffusion imaging, contributions to understanding the injury process. J Neuroradiol 2007;34(2):111; with permission.)

after AHT.[19] When cases of AHT or accidental TBI of the same Glasgow Coma Scale (GCS) score are compared, AHT groups generally have poorer outcomes. Children with moderate AHT and GCS score of 9 to 11 have a mortality risk similar to that of children with severe accidental TBI and GCS score less than 9.[20]

Compared to those with accidental TBI, children with AHT tend to be younger, are more likely to be brought in from home, and are more likely to have both apnea and seizures. Both groups are at equal risk of hypotension and hypoxemia. The ultimate cause of death in both groups is related to intracranial hypertension.[21]

Management of Abusive Head Trauma

Guidelines on the management of pediatric TBI largely stem from studies that either group accidental TBI and AHT together or exclude AHT because of its complex nature. Some clinicians suggest that AHT should be treated more aggressively than accidental TBI, specifically with more aggressive intracranial pressure (ICP) management. However, this strategy is not supported by current data.[24] Therefore, current

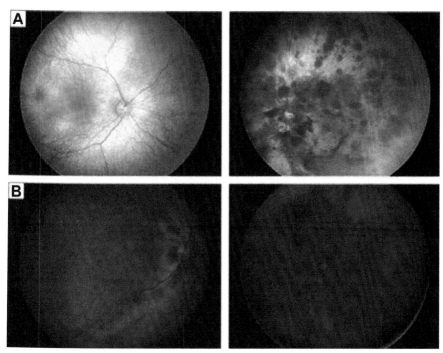

Fig. 3. (*A*) RetCam photographs of a 3-month-old boy diagnosed with AHT who subsequently died. The posterior pole and periphery showed no hemorrhages, but there were severe multilayered hemorrhages noted in the left eye, with preretinal hemorrhage layered in the inferior macula of the left eye. (*B*) RetCam photographs of a 4-month-old boy diagnosed with AHT showing bilateral severe retinal hemorrhages greater in the left eye. The hemorrhages are asymmetric, with the left side having more hemorrhages than the right, but both show multilayered retinal hemorrhages in the posterior pole and periphery. (*From* Longmuir SQ, McConnell L, Oral R, et al. Retinal hemorrhages in intubated pediatric intensive care patients. J AAPOS 2014;18(2):132; with permission.)

Table 3			
Abusive head trauma is multifactorial			
Shaking	Cervical Spine Injury	Bridging Vein Tears	Intracranial Hypertension
Blunt force	Thoracic spine injury	Subdural hematomas in the brain and spine	Hypoventilation, apnea
Impact	Hypoxic ischemic injury (especially if medical care is delayed)	Retinal hemorrhages	Coagulopathy
Acceleration-deceleration	Brain stem injury	Immature cervical ligaments and muscles in infants	Hypothermia
Diffuse axonal injury	Shearing forces	Seizures	Hypotension

Data from Refs.[19,22,23]

recommendations are to follow pediatric TBI guidelines without any cause-specific modifications (**Box 3**). Please also refer to **Table 4** regarding calculation of pediatric GCS. The pediatric GCS scale is recommended for children two years old and younger, as their verbalization cannot be assessed using adult criteria.

Preoperative planning begins in the trauma bay with initiation of vascular access, volume resuscitation as required, and ordering of blood products. Airway management must focus on first-attempt success to avoid periods of prolonged apnea, which can lead to hypoxia and hypercarbia. An ideal approach includes rapid sequence induction, and the choice of induction medications and depolarizing or nondepolarizing muscle relaxants is at the discretion of the anesthesiologist. Etomidate, although cardiac stable, is associated with potential future adrenal suppression. Ketamine also maintains blood pressure but carries a theoretic risk of increase in ICP, although this is rarely seen in clinical practice. Propofol is familiar and reduces cerebral metabolic rate but can cause transient hypotension.

For patients with severe intracranial hypertension, intermittent ventilation with low ventilator pressure may be needed to avoid the aforementioned hypercarbia and hypoxia, which may cause catastrophic increases in ICP. Cervical spine in-line stabilization is essential, even if radiographic films are normal because pediatric spine injuries may be missed on radiographs. AHT may cause significant bleeding from mechanical tearing of bridging veins and potential late injury presentation.

If the infant or child requires additional radiologic studies and is hemodynamically stable, it is helpful to obtain such studies promptly after surgery to prevent delay in diagnosing additional injuries. If the patient received an ophthalmologic examination, the anesthesiologist must know which eye was dilated preoperatively. Consider also that biomarker use to detect or predict TBI over the last decade is limited by small

---

Box 3
Summary of pediatric traumatic brain injury guidelines

- Maintain ICP <20 mm Hg.
- Maintain cerebral perfusion pressure (CPP) $\geq$40 to 50 mm Hg, and adjust target CPP ranges for age.
- Use methods to decrease the ICP while simultaneously supporting the CPP through hemodynamic support. It is not sufficient to increase blood pressure alone.
- Avoid hypoxia.
- Avoid hypercarbia.
- Reserve hyperventilation for treatment of refractory intracranial hypertension with impending brain herniation. Hyperventilation causes cerebral vasoconstriction, which may cause cerebral ischemia.
- Avoid hyperthermia.
- Consider treatment of early post-traumatic seizures.
- Elevate the head of bed.
- Use hypertonic saline, barbiturates, or decompressive craniectomy to treat intracranial hypertension. Mannitol is second line to hypertonic saline.
- Use ICP monitoring in patients with GCS score <9.

Data from Shein SL, Bell MJ, Kochanek PM, et al. Risk factors for mortality in children with abusive head trauma. J Pediatr 2012;161(4):716–22.e1; and Hardcastle N, Benzon HA, Vavilala MS. Update on the 2012 guidelines for the management of pediatric traumatic brain injury - information for the anesthesiologist. Paediatr Anaesth 2014;24(7):703–10.

Table 4
Modified Glasgow Coma Scale for young children and infants

	Pediatric	Infants	Score
Eyes	Open spontaneously	Open spontaneously	4
	React to speech	React to speech	3
	React to pain	React to pain	2
	No response	No response	1
Verbal	Smiles, appears oriented, interactive	Coos, babbles, interactive	5
	Interacts inappropriately for age	Irritable	4
	Moans	Cries to pain	3
	Irritable, inconsolable	Moans to pain	2
	No response	No response	1
Motor	Follows commands	Spontaneous movements	6
	Localizes pain	Withdraws to touch	5
	Withdraws to pain	Withdraws to pain	4
	Abnormal flexion	Abnormal flexion	3
	Extension posturing	Extensive posturing	2
	No response	No response	1

Based on Institute of Neurological Sciences NHS Greater Glasgow and Clyde. Glasgow Coma Scale: Do it this way. Available at: http://www.glasgowcomascale.org/downloads/GCS-Assessment-Aid-English.pdf?v=3. Accessed October 16, 2018.

sample size, variable practices in sample collection, inconsistent biomarker-related data elements, and disparate outcome measures. Future studies of biomarkers for pediatric TBI are needed.[25]

Prevention of Abusive Head Trauma

Several states mandate AHT education in the postnatal period, and the results have been mixed. The Safe Babies New York program taught parents about normal crying behavior, how to comfort crying babies, how to reduce caregiver frustration or anger, and about the medical impact of shaking an infant. This program showed a 47% reduction in incidence in AHT over six years.[26] However, similar programs in Pennsylvania and North Carolina showed no reduction in the overall incidence of AHT.[27,28] With continued improvements in data collection and analysis, clinicians hope to better identify high-risk groups and create more effective AHT prevention strategies.[29]

Second Victim Considerations

Child abuse cases cause significant psychological impact on clinicians, thereby creating a second victim. Second victim symptoms include anxiety, depression, confusion, loss of confidence, and sleep derangement. Each of these increase the risk of future medical errors.[30] Clinicians must recognize second victim harm and support fellow clinicians during and after treatment of child abuse.

THE PEDIATRIC TRAUMATIC BRAIN INJURY SPECTRUM: SPORTS-RELATED CONCUSSIONS

This overview thus far focuses on AHT with associated NAT as a subset of pediatric TBI. AHT involves younger children and is both acute and devastating. Sports-related mild TBI tends to affect older children, with a peak in adolescence, and represents the other end of the pediatric TBI spectrum. It is subacute with more subtle presentation and leads to potentially debilitating neurocognitive deficits. The rest of this overview focuses on sports-related TBI with associated anesthetic considerations.

Sports-related Traumatic Brain Injury in Children and Adolescents

Concussion and other forms of mild TBI constitute approximately 75% of TBI's that present per year, and mild TBI accounts for 16% of children less than ten years of age presenting for medical attention.[31,32] Although TBI in the pediatric population is most commonly caused by falls and motor vehicle accidents, approximately 1.9 million youth have sports concussion annually, and 60% to 80% of pediatric sports-related hospitalizations are a result of pediatric sports-related TBI.[33,34] Most common causes of sports-related concussion among boys include football, hockey, and lacrosse, whereas soccer, lacrosse, and basketball account for the leading causes among girls.[31,35] Between 1996 and 2010, there were more than 78,000 snow sports–related head injuries among children and adolescents.[36] The incidence of pediatric sports-related concussion is highest among the adolescent group, particularly in the 15-year-old to 19-year-old age group, and recent studies have indicated that the incidence of diagnosed pediatric sports-related concussion is increasing.[37,38]

Concussion is defined as brain injury resulting from biomechanical forces that may or may not present with loss of consciousness but leads to brief changes in mental status and neurologic function impairment in the absence of visible abnormalities on standard structural neuroimaging studies.[39] Concussion typically presents with a range of symptoms including headache, lethargy, memory impairment, cognitive deficits, dizziness, problems with balance, sleep disturbances, and psychiatric symptoms. Symptoms are generally rapid in onset and resolve within a week to ten days from injury. However, up to 30% of children with concussion have symptoms that extend beyond 28 days after injury, a phenomenon known as persistent postconcussive symptoms.[40,41]

Pathophysiology of Concussion

Although the pathophysiology of concussion is not definitively elucidated, it is known that changes in cerebrovascular homeostatis commonly occur following concussion injury and likely contribute to brain injury and brain vulnerability. Impairment of cerebral autoregulation after concussion is well established and renders the brain susceptible to injury from cerebral ischemia or hyperemia.[42] Mild to severe TBI, specifically in the pediatric population, has been shown to not only impair cerebral autoregulation; however, this impairment increases with younger age and is associated with worse six-month prognosis.[43–45] Recently, Vavilala and colleagues[46] examined cerebral autoregulation in youth who were hospitalized after sports-related mild TBI. By measuring middle cerebral artery flow velocity and cerebral autoregulation index using transcranial Doppler ultrasonography and tilt testing, the study showed that impaired cerebral autoregulation is common in sports-related TBI and occurs even when all of the patients' presenting and serial daily GCS scores were 15.[46]

Sports-related concussion in teenage athletes has been shown to result in diminished changes in cerebral flow in response to hypocapnia and hypercapnia compared with healthy controls.[47] Prolonged decreases in cerebral blood flow can continue for weeks to months after injury and correlate with persistent postconcussive symptoms.[48,49] In addition, imaging studies have shown that cerebral metabolic rates often increase after concussion, and the increased oxygen demand may further render the brain vulnerable to injury, particularly in the setting of compromised supply caused by decreased cerebral blood flow.[47,50] Increased neurotransmitter release and inflammatory cytokine expression can occur after concussion, which may lead to cytotoxic cerebral edema and diffuse axonal injury.[51,52]

Anesthesia and Surgery Following Concussion in the Pediatric Population

The effects of general anesthesia or surgery on the brain in the postconcussive period have not been well researched. However, anesthesiologists should be concerned with the potential risks that both general anesthesia and surgery may pose to postconcussive patients. For instance, volatile anesthetics may further undermine the cerebrovascular autoregulation impairment known to be present in even mild pediatric TBI. It is known that, in pediatric TBI in general, blood pressure and glucose control and maintenance of normal oxygenation and ventilation directly affect patient outcomes.[53] Hence, the so-called secondary insults commonly produced by general anesthesia and surgery, which include hypotension and decreased cerebral perfusion, hypocarbia or hypercarbia, and hyperglycemia, could potentially exacerbate concussive brain injury and delay recovery of symptoms.[54]

A recent poll of attendees of the Fall 2016 Washington State Society of Anesthesiologists meeting revealed that although 93% of providers responded that screening for concussion is important, only 5% reported that they conducted routine screening.[55] In a study conducted by Ferrari and colleagues,[56] a questionnaire was administered during the preoperative assessment to patients between the ages of five and 21 years who presented for surgical repair of orthopedic traumatic injury or nasal fracture, and who had precipitating injury within four weeks of the proposed surgery. Depending on age, at-risk patients were given either the Sport Concussion Assessment Tool (SCAT-3) or the Child Sport Concussion Assessment Tool (Child SCAT-3) to elicit self-reported symptoms of concussion. The prevalence of recent concussion diagnosed during the preoperative period for children undergoing semielective orthopedic surgery was approximately 6%. Moreover, only one in seven patients who had SCAT-3 or Child SCAT-3 scores suggestive of concussion had a preoperative diagnosis of concussion before the preoperative assessment.

A retrospective analysis identified patients who were diagnosed with concussion at the Mayo Clinic (Rochester, MN) between 2005 and 2015 who underwent a surgical procedure and anesthesia under the care of a physician anesthesiologist. Of the 1038 patients who were identified by these criteria, 93% (n = 965) had anesthesia one week after injury. Of note, 7% of patient with concussion had a delay in diagnosis of more than one week after injury, and several of these patients had undergone anesthesia before a concussion diagnosis. Of the patients who had surgery within one week after concussive injury, 5% underwent anesthesia for surgical procedures that were considered to be elective and unrelated to the concussive injury.[57]

The results of both of the studies signify that anesthesia and surgery may often confer a real and clinically significant risk of secondary insult soon after initial injury before the brain has had time to recover. Second, the studies show that a formal diagnosis of concussion is often missed, and that many patients with concussion fail to report symptoms of head injury to medical providers. Patients and families may fail to disclose these symptoms for multiple reasons, including symptoms being vague or mild and that recognition of signs of concussion are unknown, particularly when patients present in outpatient settings. In spite of official statements made by the National Football League, the American Academy of Pediatrics, and the American Academy of Neurology on recognition of concussion symptoms and return-to-play guidelines, studies show that around one-third of athletes do not recognize their symptoms as resulting from concussion.[58] Distracting injury can obscure recognition of neurocognitive symptoms. Moreover, the neurocognitive side effects of opioids administered for pain control may also cloud the observation and monitoring of cognitive dysfunction caused by concussion.[59]

Persistent Postconcussion Symptoms

Although most concussion symptoms resolve within 28 days of injury, a prospective multicenter cohort study enrolling more than 3000 patients between the ages of five and 17 years who presented with acute concussion in the emergency department revealed that almost one-third had persistent postconcussive symptoms lasting for longer than one month.[41] A retrospective case control study of 294 children presenting to a tertiary care concussion clinic identified risk factors that may result in delayed recovery from pediatric sports-related concussion. The study also found that approximately one-third of patients with concussion had persistent postconcussive symptoms beyond 28 days. Previous history of concussion, concussion injury resulting from nonhelmeted sports, female gender, presenting SCAT-2 score less than 80, SCAT-2 symptom severity score greater than 20, and previous diagnosis of attention-deficit/hyperactivity disorder were factors that predicted for concussion symptoms lasting greater than 28 days.[60] Similarly, a retrospective cohort study that evaluated children undergoing MRI for persistent symptoms after pediatric sports-related concussion identified female gender and history of previous TBI to be associated with a delayed resolution of postconcussive symptoms.[61] Although both of these studies are retrospective analyses, they provide evidence suggesting that persistent postconcussive symptoms are a relevant issue that anesthesiologists should be aware of and actively evaluate for during their assessments.

Summary of Pediatric Sports Related Concussions

Although there is no evidence to delineate optimal management of patients for semielective surgeries or provide definitive guidelines for timing of elective procedures, it is clear that anesthesiologists play a crucial role in providing optimal care for patients who have had concussion. As such, anesthesiologists may be pivotal in routine screening for risk and symptoms of concussion during preanesthesia evaluations, regardless of whether the patients carry prior diagnoses. Routine screening should include a detailed evaluation and clear, direct questioning of risk factors and concussive symptoms, which could include a modified version of the SCAT questionnaire (https://bjsm.bmj.com/content/bjsports/47/5/259.full.pdf). Screening of concussion symptoms even beyond one month after the concussion injury may be important in identifying the at-risk population. At a minimum, it may be prudent to defer elective surgeries and procedures requiring anesthesia until postconcussive symptoms have fully resolved. For nonelective procedures, the anesthetic management should be precise and follow the general principles of TBI care outlined earlier to minimize secondary insults. To effectively establish best-practice guidelines, further discussion, education on awareness, and research need to be prioritized in order to identify optimal means of screening for and managing postconcussive patients in the perioperative period (**Box 4**). Prospective studies will be critical to evaluate the effect of anesthesia and surgery on postconcussion patient outcomes.

> **Box 4**
> **Knowledge Gap Areas in Perioperative Concussion**
>
> Some potential questions regarding perioperative care of pediatric patients with concussion:
> - What do anesthesiologists know, think, and believe?
> - What is the current anesthesia practice?
> - Should anesthesiologists or surgeons screen?
> - Should anesthesiologists modify anesthesia care?
> - Should patients with concussion receive opioids at discharge?
> - What is the best anesthetic technique?
> - Should anesthesiologists delay surgery for symptomatic patients?
> - Does timing of concussion affect decision to proceed and/or anesthetic technique?
> - Should guidelines be developed for the care of concussed patients requiring elective surgery?
> - Should hemodynamic targets be different in concussion?
>
> *From* Vavilala MS, Ferrari LR, Herring SA. Perioperative care of the concussed patient: making the case for defining best anesthesia care. Anesth Analg 2017;125(3):1054; with permission.

REFERENCES

1. Leeb RT, Paulozzi LJ, Melanson C, et al. Child maltreatment surveillance uniform definitions for public health and recommended data elements version 1.0. 2008. Available at: https://www.cdc.gov/violenceprevention/pdf/CM_Surveillance-a. pdf. Accessed July 5, 2018.
2. Leeb RT, Fluke JD. Child maltreatment surveillance: enumeration, monitoring, evaluation and insight. Health Promot Chronic Dis Prev Can 2015;35(8–9): 138–40. Available at: http://www.ncbi.nlm.nih.gov/pubmed/26605561. Accessed July 5, 2018.
3. Christian CW, Block R, Committee on Child Abuse and Neglect, American Academy of Pediatrics. Abusive head trauma in infants and children. Pediatrics 2009; 123(5):1409–11.
4. US Department of Health and Human Services, Administration for Children and Families, Administration on Children Youth and Families, Children's Bureau. Child Maltreatment 2016. 2018. Available at: https://www.acf.hhs.gov/sites/default/files/ cb/cm2016.pdf. Accessed June 26, 2018.
5. Yu DTY, Ngo TL. Child abuse—a review of inflicted intraoral, esophageal, and abdominal visceral injuries. Clin Pediatr Emerg Med 2016;17(4):284–95.
6. Beers SR, Berger RP, Adelson PD. Neurocognitive outcome and serum biomarkers in inflicted versus non-inflicted traumatic brain injury in young children. J Neurotrauma 2007;24(1):97–105.
7. Ellingson KD, Leventhal JM, Weiss HB. Using hospital discharge data to track inflicted traumatic brain injury. Am J Prev Med 2008;34(4):S157–62.
8. Salehi-Had H, Brandt JD, Rosas AJ, et al. Findings in older children with abusive head injury: does shaken-child syndrome exist? Pediatrics 2006;117(5): e1039–44.
9. Fishe JN, Moffat FL. Child abuse and the law. Clin Pediatr Emerg Med 2016;17(4): 302–11.
10. Sheets LK, Leach ME, Koszewski IJ, et al. Sentinel injuries in infants evaluated for child physical abuse. Pediatrics 2013;131(4):701–7.
11. Ward MG, Ornstein A, Niec A, et al, Canadian Paediatric Society, Child and Youth Maltreatment Section. The medical assessment of bruising in suspected child maltreatment cases: a clinical perspective. Paediatr Child Health 2013;18(8):

433–42. Available at: http://www.ncbi.nlm.nih.gov/pubmed/24426797. Accessed July 3, 2018.

12. Naik-Mathuria B, Akinkuotu A, Wesson D. Role of the surgeon in non-accidental trauma. Pediatr Surg Int 2015;31(7):605–10.

13. Narain A. Skeletal manifestations of child maltreatment. Clin Pediatr Emerg Med 2016;17(4):274–83.

14. Perez-Rossello JM, McDonald AG, Rosenberg AE, et al. Absence of rickets in infants with fatal abusive head trauma and classic metaphyseal lesions. Radiology 2015;275(3):810–21.

15. Niederkrotenthaler T, Xu L, Parks SE, et al. Descriptive factors of abusive head trauma in young children—United States, 2000–2009. Child Abuse Negl 2013; 37(7):446–55.

16. Kesler H, Dias MS, Shaffer M, et al. Demographics of abusive head trauma in the Commonwealth of Pennsylvania. J Neurosurg Pediatr 2008;1(5):351–6.

17. Jenny C, Hymel KP, Ritzen A, et al. Analysis of missed cases of abusive head trauma. JAMA 1999;281(7):621.

18. Adamsbaum C, Grabar S, Mejean N, et al. Abusive head trauma: judicial admissions highlight violent and repetitive shaking. Pediatrics 2010;126(3):546–55.

19. Duhaime A-C, Durham S. Traumatic brain injury in infants: the phenomenon of subdural hemorrhage with hemispheric hypodensity ("Big Black Brain"). Prog Brain Res 2007;161:293–302.

20. Shein SL, Bell MJ, Kochanek PM, et al. Risk factors for mortality in children with abusive head trauma. J Pediatr 2012;161(4):716–22.e1.

21. Miller Ferguson N, Sarnaik A, Miles D, et al. Abusive head trauma and mortality–an analysis from an international comparative effectiveness study of children with severe traumatic brain injury. Crit Care Med 2017;45(8):1398–407.

22. Longmuir SQ, McConnell L, Oral R, et al. Retinal hemorrhages in intubated pediatric intensive care patients. J AAPOS 2014;18(2):129–33.

23. Lee JK, Brady KM, Deutsch N. The anesthesiologist's role in treating abusive head trauma. Anesth Analg 2016;122(6):1971–82.

24. Hardcastle N, Benzon HA, Vavilala MS. Update on the 2012 guidelines for the management of pediatric traumatic brain injury - information for the anesthesiologist. Paediatr Anaesth 2014;24(7):703–10.

25. Papa L, Ramia MM, Kelly JM, et al. Systematic review of clinical research on biomarkers for pediatric traumatic brain injury. J Neurotrauma 2013;30(5):324–38.

26. Dias MS, Smith K, DeGuehery K, et al. Preventing abusive head trauma among infants and young children: a hospital-based, parent education program. Pediatrics 2005;115(4):e470–7.

27. Dias MS, Rottmund CM, Cappos KM, et al. Association of a postnatal parent education program for abusive head trauma with subsequent pediatric abusive head trauma hospitalization rates. JAMA Pediatr 2017;171(3):223.

28. Zolotor AJ, Runyan DK, Shanahan M, et al. Effectiveness of a statewide abusive head trauma prevention program in North Carolina. JAMA Pediatr 2015;169(12): 1126.

29. Kelly P, Thompson JMD, Koh J, et al. Perinatal risk and protective factors for pediatric abusive head trauma: a multicenter case-control study. J Pediatr 2017; 187:240–6.e4.

30. Marmon LM, Heiss K. Improving surgeon wellness: the second victim syndrome and quality of care. Semin Pediatr Surg 2015;24:315–8.

31. Barlow KM, Crawford S, Stevenson A, et al. Epidemiology of postconcussion syndrome in pediatric mild traumatic brain injury. Pediatrics 2010;126(2):e374–81.

32. National Center for Injury Prevention and Control. Report to Congress on mild traumatic brain injury in the United States: steps to prevent a serious public health problem. Atlanta (GA): Centers for Disease Control and Prevention; 2003.

33. Bryan MA, Rowhani-Rahbar A, Comstock RD, et al. Sports- and recreation-related concussions in US youth. Pediatrics 2016;138(1) [pii:e20154635].

34. Yue JK, Winkler EA, Burke JF, et al. Pediatric sports-related traumatic brain injury in United States trauma centers. Neurosurg Focus 2016;40(4):E3.

35. Noble JM, Hesdorffer DC. Sport-related concussions: a review of epidemiology, challenges in diagnosis, and potential risk factors. Neuropsychol Rev 2013; 23(4):273–84.

36. Graves JM, Whitehill JM, Stream JO, et al. Emergency department reported head injuries from skiing and snowboarding among children and adolescents, 1996-2010. Inj Prev 2013;19(6):399–404.

37. Gessel LM, Fields SK, Collins CL, et al. Concussions among United States high school and collegiate athletes. J Athl Train 2007;42(4):495.

38. Zhang AL, Sing DC, Rugg CM, et al. The rise of concussions in the adolescent population. Orthop J Sports Med 2016;4(8). 2325967116662458.

39. McCrory P, Meeuwisse WH, Aubry M, et al. Consensus statement on concussion in sport: the 4th International Conference on Concussion in Sport held in Zurich, November 2012. Br J Sports Med 2013;47(5):250–8.

40. Eisenberg MA, Meehan WP, Mannix R. Duration and course of post-concussive symptoms. Pediatrics 2014;133(6):999–1006.

41. Zemek R, Barrowman N, Freedman SB, et al. Clinical risk score for persistent postconcussion symptoms among children with acute concussion in the ED. JAMA 2016;315(10):1014–25.

42. Obrist WD, Gennarelli TA, Segawa H, et al. Relation of cerebral blood flow to neurological status and outcome in head-injured patients. J Neurosurg 1979; 51(3):292–300.

43. Vavilala MS, Lee LA, Boddu K, et al. Cerebral autoregulation in pediatric traumatic brain injury. Pediatr Crit Care Med 2004;5(3):257–63.

44. Freeman SS, Udomphorn Y, Armstead WM, et al. Young age as a risk factor for impaired cerebral autoregulation after moderate to severe pediatric traumatic brain injury. Anesthesiology 2008;108(4):588–95.

45. Chaiwat O, Sharma D, Udomphorn Y, et al. Cerebral hemodynamic predictors of poor 6-month Glasgow Outcome Score in severe pediatric traumatic brain injury. J Neurotrauma 2009;26(5):657–63.

46. Vavilala MS, Farr CK, Watanitanon A, et al. Early changes in cerebral autoregulation among youth hospitalized after sports-related traumatic brain injury. Brain Inj 2018;32(2):269–75.

47. Len T, Neary J. Cerebrovascular pathophysiology following mild traumatic brain injury. Clin Physiol Funct Imaging 2011;31(2):85–93.

48. Bonne O, Gilboa A, Louzoun Y, et al. Cerebral blood flow in chronic symptomatic mild traumatic brain injury. Psychiatry Res Neuroimaging 2003;124(3):141–52.

49. Maugans TA, Farley C, Altaye M, et al. Pediatric sports-related concussion produces cerebral blood flow alterations. Pediatrics 2012;129(1):28–37.

50. Lovell MR, Pardini JE, Welling J, et al. Functional brain abnormalities are related to clinical recovery and time to return-to-play in athletes. Neurosurgery 2007; 61(2):352–60.

51. Patterson ZR, Holahan MR. Understanding the neuroinflammatory response following concussion to develop treatment strategies. Front Cell Neurosci 2012; 6:58.

52. Choe MC, Babikian T, DiFiori J, et al. A pediatric perspective on concussion pathophysiology. Curr Opin Pediatr 2012;24(6):689–95.

53. Kannan N, Ramaiah R, Vavilala MS. Pediatric neurotrauma. Int J Crit Illn Inj Sci 2014;4(2):131.

54. Vavilala MS, Ferrari LR, Herring SA. Perioperative care of the concussed patient: making the case for defining best anesthesia care. Anesth Analg 2017;125(3): 1053–5.

55. NIH NIONDAS. Pediatric Concussion Workshop. 2016, October 13-14. Available at: https://meetings.ninds.nih.gov/Home/General/15077. Accessed November 18, 2016.

56. Ferrari LR, O'Brien MJ, Taylor AM, et al. Concussion in pediatric surgical patients scheduled for time-sensitive surgical procedures. J Concussion 2017;1. 2059700217704775.

57. Abcejo AS, Savica R, Lanier WL, et al. Exposure to surgery and anesthesia after concussion due to mild traumatic brain injury. Mayo Clin Proc 2017;92(7): 1042–52.

58. McCrea M, Hammeke T, Olsen G, et al. Unreported concussion in high school football players: implications for prevention. Clin J Sport Med 2004;14(1):13–7.

59. Pinchefsky E, Dubrovsky AS, Friedman D, et al. Part II—Management of pediatric post-traumatic headaches. Pediatr Neurol 2015;52(3):270–80.

60. Miller JH, Gill C, Kuhn EN, et al. Predictors of delayed recovery following pediatric sports-related concussion: a case-control study. J Neurosurg Pediatr 2016;17(4): 491–6.

61. Bonow RH, Friedman SD, Perez FA, et al. Prevalence of abnormal magnetic resonance imaging findings in children with persistent symptoms after pediatric sports-related concussion. J Neurotrauma 2017;34(19):2706–12.

The Lifetime Effects of Injury
Postintensive Care Syndrome and Posttraumatic Stress Disorder

Meghan B. Lane-Fall, MD, MSHP[a,b,*], Catherine M. Kuza, MD[c], Samir Fakhry, MD[d], Lewis J. Kaplan, MD[e]

KEYWORDS

• PICS • Trauma • PTSD • Outcomes

KEY POINTS

- Postintensive care syndrome (PICS) is a heterogeneous syndrome marked by the physical, cognitive, and mental health impairments experienced by critical care survivors.
- PICS is a syndrome that bears significant human and health care costs. Additional research is needed to identify risk factors and diagnostic, preventative, and treatment strategies for PICS.
- Trauma intensive care unit patients are particularly vulnerable to posttraumatic stress disorder, which shares some of the adverse long-term consequences of PICS and requires additional research into effective preventative and management strategies.

Disclosures: The authors have no disclosures.
[a] Department of Anesthesiology and Critical Care, Perelman School of Medicine, University of Pennsylvania, 423 Guardian Drive, 309 Blockley Hall, Philadelphia, PA 19104, USA; [b] Leonard Davis Institute of Health Economics, University of Pennsylvania, 3641 Locust Walk # 210, Philadelphia, PA 19104, USA; [c] Department of Anesthesiology and Critical Care, Keck School of Medicine of the University of Southern California, Los Angeles County Health System, 1450 San Pablo Street, Suite 3600, Los Angeles, CA 90033, USA; [d] Department of Surgery, Synergy Surgicalists, Inc, Reston Hospital Center, 1850 Town Center Parkway Suite 309, Reston, VA 20190, USA; [e] Surgical Services, Department of Surgery, Division of Trauma, Surgical Critical Care and Emergency Surgery, Hospital of the University of Pennsylvania, Veteran's Administration Medical Center, Corporal Michael J Crescenz VA Medical Center, Perelman School of Medicine, University of Pennsylvania, 3900 Woodland Avenue, Philadelphia, PA 19104, USA
* Corresponding author. Department of Anesthesiology and Critical Care, 309 Blockley Hall, Philadelphia, PA 19104-4865.
E-mail address: meghan.lanefall@uphs.upenn.edu

Anesthesiology Clin 37 (2019) 135–150
https://doi.org/10.1016/j.anclin.2018.09.012
1932-2275/19/© 2018 Elsevier Inc. All rights reserved.

anesthesiology.theclinics.com

INTRODUCTION

Over the past 30 years, intensive care unit (ICU) service utilization has experienced sustained growth.[1,2] Concomitantly, ICU patient survival has improved, leading to a growing population of survivors, many of whom suffer from ICU-related complications into their convalesence.[3–5] Increasing awareness of ICU survivor disabilities has crystallized the constellation of related signs and symptoms as the postintensive care syndrome (PICS).[6] This article explores PICS in detail, including the pathophysiology, prevention, diagnosis, management, and unknown aspects driving current investigation. Special attention is devoted to the part of PICS associated with psychiatric sequelae. Polytrauma patients admitted to the hospital are particularly vulnerable to developing disorders such as depression, anxiety, and posttraumatic stress disorder (PTSD).[7] Those requiring ICU care are at a greater risk of developing psychiatric disorders and make up a subset of critically ill patients expected to have worsened trajectories of quality of life (QOL).[8] Because of the high incidence of PTSD and its adverse consequences in trauma patients, persisting up to 14 years postinjury, including impaired QOL and an inability to return to work or baseline physical function,[7–10] this article discusses this topic in greater depth. Although the primary focus is on ICU survivors, the impact of PICS on family members (PICS-F) is also explored.[6]

DEFINITION AND PATHOPHYSIOLOGY OF POSTINTENSIVE CARE SYNDROME

PICS was defined at a stakeholder consensus meeting in 2010 as a tripartite syndrome involving (1) physical, (2) cognitive, and (3) mental health impairment in ICU survivors.[6] Each of these elements has been previously described as a unique, and sometimes unavoidable, complication of intensive care.[11] For example, patients with long ICU lengths of stay (LOS) are less likely to be discharged home, with a substantial proportion being discharged to facilities providing inpatient rehabilitation, skilled nursing, or long-term acute care.[12] Prolonged functional impairment[11] and delayed return to work[13] are some of the untoward and potentially avoidable experiences reported by critical illness survivors before the codification of PICS as a formal diagnosis.[6,14]

Despite increasing recognition of the impairments that follow critical illness, PICS demonstrates a variable penetrance across ICU survivor populations. A variety of PICS triggers have been identified (**Fig. 1**), including immobility, delirium, inadequate or inappropriate sedation or analgesia, disordered communication, and inadequate or absent family communication or support. This article explores PICS diagnostic elements and identifies opportunities for linking triggers to potential therapeutic intervention.

Physical Impairment

After prolonged critical illness, compared with healthy counterparts, generalized muscular weakness is common and potential risk factors have been identified (**Table 1**).[15,16] Unsurprisingly, the most pronounced weakness occurs in those with the longest ICU LOS.[12] Skeletal muscle seems disproportionately affected compared with smooth muscle, regardless of the adequacy or route of nutritional support.[17–19] Accordingly, this observation has also been termed ICU-acquired weakness.[17,20] Recent work links persistent inflammation and immunosuppression to prolonged ICU LOS through a hypermetabolic state called persistent inflammation, infection, and catabolism syndrome (PIICS).[21] PIICS seems related to the activity of suppressor macrophages and lymphoid elements, and causes a state of multiple organ dysfunction that can prolong or prevent recovery.[22] Although weakness is part of PIICS, it seems to have different underpinnings than the weakness that accompanies PICS.

Triggers

PICS

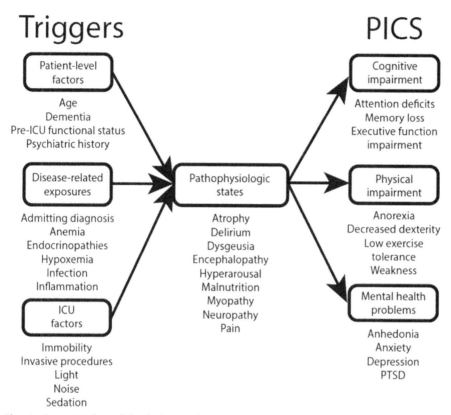

Patient-level factors

Age
Dementia
Pre-ICU functional status
Psychiatric history

Disease-related exposures

Admitting diagnosis
Anemia
Endocrinopathies
Hypoxemia
Infection
Inflammation

ICU factors

Immobility
Invasive procedures
Light
Noise
Sedation

Pathophysiologic states

Atrophy
Delirium
Dysgeusia
Encephalopathy
Hyperarousal
Malnutrition
Myopathy
Neuropathy
Pain

Cognitive impairment

Attention deficits
Memory loss
Executive function
impairment

Physical impairment

Anorexia
Decreased dexterity
Low exercise
tolerance
Weakness

Mental health problems

Anhedonia
Anxiety
Depression
PTSD

Fig. 1. Conceptual model relating various triggers to pathophysiologic states that are thought to precede the development of PICS.

PICS-related weakness is quantifiable using nerve conduction analysis, muscle biopsy, dynamic strength measurement, and endurance testing.[20,23] No assay demonstrates superiority in guiding therapy or predicting outcome. Related to this, less quantifiable decreases in oropharyngeal muscle strength appear as new onset

Table 1	
Putative causes of the weakness associated with critical illness	
Potential Causative Factor	**Causes of Associated Weakness**
Glucocorticoid administration	
Glucocorticoid-like effects of other agents • Antibiotics	
Immobility	Atrophy, loss of muscle mass
Hypermetabolism driven by high catecholamine tone	Loss of muscle mass
Axial skeletal muscle catabolism (fuel for gluconeogenesis during periods of inadequate nutritional support)	Loss of muscle mass
Peripheral demyelination	Nerve dysfunction
Polyneuropathy of critical illness	Nerve dysfunction

dysphagia, which is identified in a binary fashion rather than as reduced amplitude. Other surrogates are prolonged mechanical ventilation[23] and tracheostomy placement. Current measures of respiratory muscle strength and endurance are less robust than is optimal, and surrogate measures are plagued by a lack of precision due to overlap with comorbid processes and clinical pathways that use time metrics rather than metrics rooted in functional assessment.

Cognitive Impairment

The ability to manage one's affairs, both financial and personal, is crucial in the transition to independent living. Although such a transition does rely in part on the physical capacity to engage in the activities of daily living, cognitive impairment may preclude it.[24] In PICS, ICU survivor neurocognitive inquiries show that memory[25,26] and executive function[25,27] are substantially affected, and that decrements in attention,[26] processing speed,[26,27] and visuospatial orientation commonly occur.[27] These findings are in part actionable because memory aids and retraining regimens may mitigate such deficiencies both temporarily and permanently. However, there is little to offer for rapid recovery from impaired executive function. Therefore, there is a clear imperative to understand the triggers for such a debilitating event.

Delirium seems to be a key driver of post-ICU cognitive dysfunction and is better understood in terms of initiation and mitigation.[28] For this reason, substantial efforts are being undertaken to minimize or reduce exposures known to be associated with delirium (ie, benzodiazepine administration, polypharmacy, and oversedation).[29–31] The elderly population seems to be especially vulnerable to developing delirium. Recent inquiries demonstrate that delirium is associated with subsequent depression or anxiety.[32] In addition to adversely affecting virtually all care metrics, delirium may be associated with subsequent depression or anxiety.[32–36]

Mental Health Impairment

Psychiatric symptoms or disorders experienced by ICU survivors notably include anxiety, depression, and stress disorders.[8,10,37,38] In-hospital symptom occurrence increases the risk of postdischarge psychiatric sequelae, physical impairment, and decreased rehabilitation participation. The societal impact is measured in increased disability time, health care costs, financial strain, mortality rates, and potentially avoidable readmission.[39,40]

Despite previous beliefs that the critically ill do not recall ICU events, objective data present a disturbing picture of survivors plagued by undesirable memories. This potentially disabling consequence affects up to 88% of ICU survivors.[41] Indeed, therapeutic sedation to abrogate the recall phenomenon was once lauded. However, uninterrupted sedation and higher levels of sedation are strongly associated with increased ventilator days, infection, delirium, ICU and hospital LOS, and health care costs.[42] To decrease adverse events, sedation practices have evolved in favor of intermittent or minimal sedation.[42]

Unanticipated consequences of this approach may be inappropriate processing of care that was painful, unanticipated, or frightening when patients are partially sedated and not fully awake. For example, endotracheal suctioning during mechanical ventilation may lead to substantial air hunger, high catecholamine tone, anxiety, agitation, and terror. These feelings may be magnified in the setting of upper extremity restraint use for therapeutic device maintenance. Inadequate or inappropriate timing or dosing for sedation or analgesia may enable intrusive memories because the patient is inadequately prepared for an event, which leads to fear, pain, anxiety, or inappropriate interpretation of the required care event. Accordingly, required care episodes may be instead incorporated as intrusive memories[43] that surface as night terrors or nightmares, even after discharge. The tension between having an interactive patient and a comfortable patient may have, at least in part, created this aspect of PICS in an inadvertent fashion.

Sleep disorders, associated with days to weeks spent in the ICU, may result from the disruption of normal sleep–wake cycles. ICU-initiated deranged sleep–wake cycles may persist after discharge, manifesting as sleep disorders, fatigue, depression, and impaired coping mechanisms. Insomnia and other sleep disorders are common in ICU survivors[44] and they may be an initial clue that a patient is having ICU-related complications, such as PICS.

It is unsurprising that survivors may have difficulty returning to their preillness baseline. Survivors may experience personality abnormalities, difficulties with social relationships, reduced QOL,[16] and disordered appetite, as well as cognitive abnormalities. Related to this, a substantial proportion of patients never return to gainful employment.[13] This is, in many ways, anticipated and offers a specific target for inquiry and intervention given the increasing burden of health care finances for postdischarge and readmission care. There is a clearly identified opportunity to address unmet patient care needs because most PICS patients are unidentified, miscategorized, or receive care focused on a single aspect of the syndrome instead of in a global fashion. A notable exception is the injured patient population in whom directed attention has occurred to readily identify PTSD, a diagnosis whose features overlap in part with PICS.

POSTTRAUMATIC STRESS DISORDER AFTER INJURY

Originally described in war veterans, PTSD has been described in diverse populations (eg, domestic or sexual abuse victims or witnesses, patients who have cancer, family members or caretakers of disabled patients).[37] PTSD may occur after an actual or perceived event that threatens either life or perception of safety. PTSD symptoms include depressed cognition and mood; abnormal arousal and reactivity; avoidance of inciting event triggers; event reexperiencing, including flashbacks; and/or intrusive thoughts or memories.[45] Symptom persistence for more than 1 month establishes a clinical diagnosis of acute PTSD, and a duration of 3 months cements chronic PTSD.[45] PTSD has an especially high prevalence in critically ill polytrauma patients and is associated with injury severity and nature, pain, total LOS, and complications.[38] PTSD adversely affects long-term outcomes, augments care costs, and impairs return to functional independence.[46] The impact of PTSD on outcome may persist for 10 years postinjury.[10,47] Thus, it is crucial to develop and implement strategies to prevent and mitigate PTSD after trauma.

Such strategies aim to provide patient-centered health care and tailor treatment to individual needs while streamlining care coordination during transitions from hospital to rehabilitation center and then to outpatient and community settings.[9] Although ideal, this is rarely the reality after injury.[9] In particular, with transport to level 1 regional resource centers for the most severely injured, patients may receive care remote from where they live and have family support. The emphasis on physical injury management may divert attention from the psychological impact of both injury and care. Reintegration into the community of origin may occur only during rehabilitation or convalescence, leading to suboptimal information sharing during transitions of care.[9]

Prevalence

PTSD prevalence in ICU patients spans 10% to 39%, with symptom persistence up to 14 years postdischarge underpinning chronic impairment.[37,48] Acute PTSD prevalence in adult burn survivors is 20% to 45%. In adult trauma patients, the prevalence increases to 60%.[8,38]

Risk Factors

Injury severity, age, and gender do not seem to influence psychiatric outcomes post-injury, whereas being the victim of assault increases PTSD likelihood.[48,49] Risk factors for postinjury PTSD derived from meta-analyses include prior injury, prior PTSD, family history of psychiatric illness, postinjury life stressors, inadequate social support, and periinjury dysfunctional emotional content.[50-52] Other potential risk factors include injury characteristics, care intensity, ICU LOS, mechanical ventilation duration, and a non–home discharge disposition.[53] Postinjury PTSD reduces the likelihood of return to baseline function and independence.[54] Although not extensively studied, genetic factors may influence posttrauma PTSD genesis.[55] The gene encoding for pituitary adenylate cyclase-activating polypeptide receptor (ADCYAP1R1) may influence PTSD development after trauma through a polymorphism-mediated mechanism. One trial demonstrated that this polymorphism presence may portend a greater benefit of early psychological intervention.[56] Although direct ties remain to be elucidated, it seems that there may be a genetic biomarker for PTSD risk, as well as likelihood of interventions success. At present, no durable clinical recommendation may be established but this domain merits further research.

Course and Impact

One study divided postinjury PTSD subjects into 3 groups depending on their PTSD course: rapid remitting (<5 months, 56%), slow remitting (>5 months, 27%), and non-remitting (>12 months, 17%).[57] Patients who are undiagnosed or untreated, have an increased risk of chronic PTSD and its untoward sequelae.

Prevention and Treatment

In-hospital psychiatric screening and intervention

There are limited data on the efficacy of in-hospital prevention and treatment strategies other than cognitive behavioral therapy (CBT), a psychosocial intervention that helps reorient cognition patterns, as well as thoughts, behaviors, and emotional responses, through problem-solving and coping strategies.[49,58,59] In a 209-subject study of CBT deployed in an ICU, increased QOL and decreased PTSD symptoms and diagnosis seemed related to the intervention.[8] Clearly, such an intervention is resource-intensive and not necessarily generalizable but offers some hope for PTSD mitigation in the at-risk postinjury patient population.

Peer support groups

Peer support groups are voluntary collections of self-identified individuals who share empathy, advice, awareness, and emotional support oriented along the lines of a particular disease entity or diagnosis. Such groups benefit patients with a host of disorders, including cancer, coronary disease, obesity, burn victims, and substance-abuse.[60-64] The groups may be similarly useful for PTSD as well as PICS.[65,66] These groups may also help participants gain access or learn about available resources that enable recovery.[60,66] As such, incorporating CBT into postinjury peer support settings may be of benefit.[55,67] Additionally, peer support groups may serve as the sole recovery resource for patients who distrust organized medical practice and mental health practitioners in particular; these 2 characteristics have been suggested to be prevalent in those with postinjury PTSD and in injured combat veterans.[68,69] Based on low cost, ease of intervention, and putative success, alternative methods to provide peer support should be articulated and deployed for those living remotely from a major medical institution and a large body of similar survivors. It is likely that this is an under-explored domain of telemedical support that may be leveraged using a social media platform.

Psychiatric first aid and nursing psychiatric interventions

In the wake of the September 11 attacks and subsequent violent extremism events, psychiatric first-aid became publicly important as a means to mitigate anxiety and stress around such events. Such aid may be conveniently grouped into on-scene im-mediate, in-hospital, and aftercare. A formal plan to render such aid uses either trained bystanders, first-responders, or mental health professionals to provide rapid care and identify those who may benefit from more sustained aid. There is international consensus that early psychiatric first aid is beneficial after a disaster or major trauma. This intervention may help build resilience and allay anxiety and emotional distress around the index event and perhaps subsequent ones as well. Major impediments to universal deployment include but are not limited to (1) lack of a trained workforce, (2) on-scene provider safety, (3) provider transit to the scene, (4) credentialing within the medical facility, and (5) funding for aftercare.

Trauma-focused psychological interventions and cognitive behavioral therapy

CBT is a first-line intervention for established PTSD. Maladaptive behaviors and cogni-tion are thought to play a role in PTSD persistence and may be uniquely vulnerable to remedy using CBT techniques.[59] Benefits of postinjury CBT to treat PTSD seem dura-ble over a 6-month time frame.[70] Importantly, trauma-focused (as opposed to general) CBT may be coupled with eye movement desensitization and reprocessing therapy to improve outcome.[71] These coupled interventions are recommended as first-line ther-apy by the United Kingdom National Institute of Health and Clinical Excellence.[71]

Pharmacologic interventions

Pharmacologic adjuncts may augment other PTSD interventions.[72–77] The pathophys-iology of PTSD includes dysregulation of the hypothalamic-pituitary-adrenal axis and, specifically, serotonin and norepinephrine.[72] Two small, randomized controlled trials evaluated the role of hydrocortisone as PTSD prophylaxis within 12 hours of injury and noted lower 3-month PTSD symptoms; these findings have not been well embraced.[49,74] On the other hand, there is a clear role for serotonin norepinephrine re-uptake inhibitors (SNRIs) and selective serotonin reuptake inhibitors (SSRIs) with paroxetine and sertraline being the principal US Food and Drug Administration (FDA)-approved therapeutics.[72,73] Patients with debilitating symptoms that preclude psychotherapy participation may benefit from an SSRI or SNRI to facilitate trauma-focused psychotherapy.[58] Not all patients will respond to SNRI or SSRI therapy,[72] and there is no uniform metric for agent selection. Evidence supports venlafaxine, ser-traline, fluoxetine, and paroxetine over other agents in the SSRI or SNRI class for established PTSD management.[74] There is no evidence supporting the use of SSRI or SNRI in preventing PTSD.[49,57,78]

Although tricyclic antidepressants and monoamine oxidase inhibitors have been suggested to be second-line pharmacologic agents, most do not improve symptoms. Unfortunately, agents demonstrating clinical benefit are encumbered with robust adverse effects.[72] No data support using anticonvulsants, benzodiazepines, or anti-psychotics for therapy or prevention.[49,58,72] Although prazosin is not recommended as a monotherapy,[73] it has the potential to be a useful adjuvant agent[58] and may be efficacious in those with concurrent sleep disturbance, traumatic brain injury (TBI), or substance abuse disorders.[73,74] Mirtazapine and eszopiclone may also serve in an adjunctive capacity.[74] Ketamine, gabapentin, and cannabinoid receptor agonists are being investigated for use in PTSD.[49,74] Recently, the FDA has approved the limited and clinically supervised use of 3,4-Methylenedioxymethamphetamine in conjunction with psychotherapy for PTSD therapy.[76]

Trauma support network or collaborative care

The American Trauma Society developed the Trauma Survivors' Network (TSN) to prevent long-term sequelae of injury (including but not exclusively PTSD) through early identification and intervention.[79] The TSN program consists of (1) a self-help class (NextSteps); (2) a peer support program; (3) early access to information and education; and (4) an interactive Web site with social networking, providing education, information, and resources. TSN training and coordination embraces a multi-professional approach. Major obstacles to implementing TSN programs include understaffing, high start-up cost, and inadequate training time allocation. Early evidence of program deployment is promising, with improved outcomes and decreased PTSD symptoms.[7,80] Polytrauma survivors may have PTSD from their injuries and PICS related to ICU care, rendering PICS prevention and treatment equally important.

PREVENTION AND TREATMENT OF POSTINTENSIVE CARE SYNDROME

Unfortunately, most PICS-focused interventions (when PICS is recognized) are reactive and undertaken after acute care is completed. During the inpatient stay, a variety of mitigation strategies are proffered to reduce PICS incidence and penetrance. The ABCDE bundle, which is used to decrease ICU delirium,[30,81] has recently been expanded to the ABCDEFGH bundle to mitigate PICS development, and improve outcomes and care transitions (**Table 2**).[82] The bundles focus on mechanical ventilation liberation, which entails minimizing sedation, and daily awakening and spontaneous breathing trials. Delirium screening and prevention, early mobilization, and familial involvement are also highlighted.

Table 2
Bundled interventions to prevent postintensive care syndrome and improve patient outcomes in the intensive care unit, organized according to the mnemonic ABCDEFGH

A	Airway management
B	Breathing trials
C	Coordination of care Communication
D	Delirium assessment
E	Early mobility
F	Family involvement Follow-up referrals Functional reconciliation
G	Good handoff communication
H	Handout materials on PICS and PICS-F

From Harvey MA, Davidson JE. Postintensive care syndrome: right care, right now...and later. Crit Care Med 2016;44(2):384; with permission.

Few studies control for the intensity or presence of bedside physical therapy (PT). Despite firmly held preconceived notions, PT is an integral aspect of ICU recovery, even in mechanically ventilated patients.[83] Because it remains unclear whether there is a single or multiple interactive triggers for weakness, the authors remain uncertain how best to engage in prevention. Current therapies focus on mitigation rather than prevention and require active patient participation in PT regimens of varying intensities as allowed by patient condition and facility resources, including staffing. Some facilities routinely engage the patient's family members in bedside activities, including PT (range of motion, massage, and assisted ambulation). Nonetheless, weakness prevents survivors from rapidly returning to their preillness activities; including intimacy, work, childcare, and even self-care. The permanency and natural history of this specific kind of weakness awaits further study but will be difficult to discern because substantial weakness is generally met with in-patient or out-patient PT, and has been infrequently linked to PICS. Similarly, specific studies, such as electromyography and nerve conduction velocity testing, are often not performed or they are linked to a concomitant disorder (eg, stroke, injury) instead of PICS.

Although such bundled plans seem ideal, there are challenges to their execution, including adequate staffing of nurses, physical therapists, pharmacists, and nutritionists. Minimizing sedation may not be possible in all patients (eg, those with an open body cavity or acute respiratory distress syndrome). Additionally, some patients cannot participate in PT due to stroke, TBI, or hemodynamic instability. Therefore, the ability to engage in PICS mitigation strategies varies greatly on patient-related and hospital-related factors. Recent data suggest that optimal outcomes for care occur with nurse-to-patient staffing ratios of less than 1 to 1.9 and in an ICU that has significant transactive memory among team members.[84] Such an ICU has a stable nursing core with little turnover and seems to be supported by having a focused type of patient within the ICU, at least for those with injury.[85] Moreover, in 1 robust study, being cared for within the parent ICU by a multiprofessional team instead of being a boarder in another ICU while being cared for by that same team seemed to strongly affect the occurrence of delirium.[86] The impact of geographic care was not assessed in this study but may be germane with regard to PICS, especially with regard to prevention, as well as post-ICU identification, of PICS.

Few inquiries have investigated the role of social and family support systems in the quest to return to health in PICS patients. Moreover, even in a well-constructed state-specific critical care collaboration focused on quality improvement initiatives, nearly 80% of the multiprofessional members have no discussion at their institution about PICS, fewer than 15% have a formal plan for identification or mitigation, and negligibly few have a support group for survivors or families.[87] Although dramatic, it is unsurprising because, until recently, PICS was not regarded as a unique syndrome but was identified by its component parts as stand-alone elements that were not linked together in a diagnostic or therapeutic construct.

In articulating PICS treatment strategies, one must note that syndrome signs and symptoms, and therefore treatments, are distributed over time and across care settings. For this reason, careful consideration must be given to the care transitions that ICU survivors and their families experience. Transitions from ICU to ward, and from hospital ward to home, or other discharge destinations, are associated with medication errors,[88] patient and family dissatisfaction, and feelings of abandonment.[89] After hospital discharge, patients may present to primary care providers who are unfamiliar with any aspect of PICS. Poor electronic health record interoperability between health systems may interrupt information flow between inpatient and outpatient providers. This particular disconnection represents a barrier to seamless care that meets patients' and families' needs throughout recovery from critical illness. ICU follow-up clinics have been used in a small number of institutions to improve continuity but these clinics have not demonstrated clear gains in patient-centered outcomes.

It is during structured handoffs that elements influencing PICS may be reasonably addressed. Departures from usual medications administration and unusual environmental cues, including sights, sounds, smells and sensations, all contribute to delirium promotion. Structured handoffs that account for elements such as medications, daily schedules, music or television preferences, language preferences, nickname desires, and temperature preferences could help avoid delirium and the cognitive dysfunction that follows it. Data that such interventions have merit are lacking but interventions such as structured handoffs are consistent with what is known about PICS and are logically aligned with mitigation efforts.

POSTINTENSIVE CARE SYNDROME IN FAMILY MEMBERS

Multiple studies document that PICS affects family members as well as patients.[90] This condition is known as PICS-F. Depression, anxiety, and PTSD are common in family members of ICU survivors, whereas depression is predominately associated with family members whose loved one died. Family members may also experience a decreased QOL, which may be due to factors such as a lack of social and emotional support, stress of caring for a critically ill patient, financial strain due to health care costs, and an inability to return to work due for a myriad of reasons.[91,92] One review identified that 20% of ICU patient family members had to quit their job. Additionally, 29% of ICU patients could not get their jobs back and 31% depleted their family financial savings.[93] At a time when the burden on health care systems continues to increase, driving the need for earlier and seemingly more aggressive discharges to nonacute care facilities, as well as home, mitigating the impact of PICS on families merits careful evaluation.

FUTURE DIRECTIONS

The future of PICS will be defined by the discovery of new metrics for risk assessment that lead to more rapid detection and surveillance tools. At present, there are no genomic, metabolomic, or proteomic markers to generate a risk profile. Unlike acute kidney injury in which there are a variety of biomarkers, and a cell cycle arrest rubric to explain the findings at different stages, PICS is devoid of such underpinning knowledge. Furthermore, because there is no current database definition that reliably identifies patients at risk for or who have the syndrome, epidemiologic data about the extent and consequences of PICS are lacking. The primary focus should be on understanding syndrome triggers so that it may be prevented instead of managed in a reactive fashion.

Additional exploration should elucidate how to support ICU survivors throughout recovery. Patients typically progress from ICU to a ward or step-down unit, and then are discharged home or to another facility. Each transition presents an opportunity for vital information to be lost, or for care plans to become derailed. In other settings, nurse practitioners help patients and their families navigate the transition from hospital to home.[94] An analogous approach, with or without ICU follow-up clinics, has the potential to improve outcomes for ICU survivors.

SUMMARY

PICS is a heterogeneous syndrome marked by physical, cognitive, and mental health impairments experienced after surviving critical illness. Although recognition of this syndrome is increasing, additional research is needed to understand patient-level and organization-level risk factors, and effective prevention, diagnosis, and treatment strategies. In a parallel fashion, periinjury PTSD shares similar system and management features, appropriately coupling efforts at managing both syndromes in a combined system-based approach.

REFERENCES

1. Halpern NA, Pastores SM. Critical care medicine in the United States 2000-2005: an analysis of bed numbers, occupancy rates, payer mix, and costs. Crit Care Med 2010;38(1):65–71.
2. Halpern NA, Pastores SM, Greenstein RJ. Critical care medicine in the United States 1985-2000: an analysis of bed numbers, use, and costs. Crit Care Med 2004;32(6):1254–9.
3. Zilberberg MD, Shorr AF. Prolonged acute mechanical ventilation and hospital bed utilization in 2020 in the United States: Implications for budgets, plant and personnel planning. BMC Health Serv Res 2008;8:242.
4. Iwashyna TJ. Survivorship will be the defining challenge of critical care in the 21st century. Ann Intern Med 2010;153(3):204–5.
5. Iwashyna TJ, Cooke CR, Wunsch H, et al. Population burden of long-term survivorship after severe sepsis in Older Americans. J Am Geriatr Soc 2012;60(6): 1070–7.
6. Needham DM, Davidson J, Cohen H, et al. Improving long-term outcomes after discharge from intensive care unit: Report from a stakeholders' conference. Crit Care Med 2012;40(2):502–9.
7. Zatzick D, Jurkovich G, Rivara FP, et al. A randomized stepped care intervention trial targeting posttraumatic stress disorder for surgically hospitalized injury survivors. Ann Surg 2013;257(3):390–9.
8. Peris A, Bonizzoli M, Iozzelli D, et al. Early intra-intensive care unit psychological intervention promotes recovery from post traumatic stress disorders, anxiety and depression symptoms in critically ill patients. Crit Care 2011;15(1):R41.
9. Zatzick D, Russo J, Thomas P, et al. Patient-centered care transitions after injury hospitalization: a comparative effectiveness trial. Psychiatry 2018;1–17.
10. Soberg HL, Bautz-Holter E, Finset A, et al. Physical and mental health 10 years after multiple trauma: a prospective cohort study. J Trauma Acute Care Surg 2015;78(3):628–33.
11. Desai SV, Law TJ, Needham DM. Long-term complications of critical care. Crit Care Med 2011;39(2):371–9.
12. Unroe M, Kahn JM, Carson SS, et al. One-year trajectories of care and resource utilization for recipients of prolonged mechanical ventilation: a cohort study. Ann Intern Med 2010;153(3):167–75.
13. Myhren H, Ekeberg O, Stokland O. Health-related quality of life and return to work after critical illness in general intensive care unit patients: a 1-year follow-up study. Crit Care Med 2010;38(7):1554–61.
14. Elliott D, Davidson JE, Harvey MA, et al. Exploring the scope of post–intensive care syndrome therapy and care: engagement of non–critical care providers and survivors in a second stakeholders meeting. Crit Care Med 2014;42(12): 2518–26.

15. Bemis-Dougherty AR, Smith JM. What follows survival of critical illness? Physical therapists' management of patients with post-intensive care syndrome. Phys Ther 2013;93(2):179–85.

16. Herridge MS, Cheung AM, Tansey CM, et al. One-year outcomes in survivors of the acute respiratory distress syndrome. N Engl J Med 2003;348(8):683–93.

17. Friedrich O, Reid MB, Van den Berghe G, et al. The sick and the weak: neuropathies/myopathies in the critically ill. Physiol Rev 2015;95(3):1025–109.

18. Needham DM, Dinglas VD, Bienvenu OJ, et al. One year outcomes in patients with acute lung injury randomised to initial trophic or full enteral feeding: prospective follow-up of EDEN randomised trial. BMJ 2013;346:f1532.

19. Aare S, Ochala J, Norman HS, et al. Mechanisms underlying the sparing of masticatory versus limb muscle function in an experimental critical illness model. Physiol Genomics 2011;43(24):1334–50.

20. Schweickert WD, Hall J. ICU-acquired weakness. Chest 2007;131(5):1541–9.

21. Gentile LF, Cuenca AG, Efron PA, et al. Persistent inflammation and immunosuppression: a common syndrome and new horizon for surgical intensive care. J Trauma Acute Care Surg 2012;72(6):1491–501.

22. Nomellini V, Kaplan LJ, Sims CA, et al. Chronic critical illness and persistent inflammation: what can we learn from the elderly, injured, septic, and malnourished? Shock 2018;49(1):4–14.

23. Kress JP, Hall JB. ICU-acquired weakness and recovery from critical illness. N Engl J Med 2014;370(17):1626–35.

24. Hopkins RO, Jackson JC. Long-term neurocognitive function after critical illness. Chest 2006;130(3):869–78.

25. Mikkelsen ME, Christie JD, Lanken PN, et al. The adult respiratory distress syndrome cognitive outcomes study: long-term neuropsychological function in survivors of acute lung injury. Am J Respir Crit Care Med 2012;185(12):1307–15.

26. Hopkins RO, Weaver LK, Pope D, et al. Neuropsychological sequelae and impaired health status in survivors of severe acute respiratory distress syndrome. Am J Respir Crit Care Med 1999;160(1):50–6.

27. Larson MJ, Weaver LK, Hopkins RO. Cognitive sequelae in acute respiratory distress syndrome patients with and without recall of the intensive care unit. J Int Neuropsychol Soc 2007;13(4):595–605.

28. Pandharipande PP, Girard TD, Jackson JC, et al. Long-term cognitive impairment after critical illness. N Engl J Med 2013;369(14):1306–16.

29. Hopkins RO, Spuhler VJ. Strategies for promoting early activity in critically ill mechanically ventilated patients. AACN Adv Crit Care 2009;20(3):277–89.

30. Pandharipande P, Banerjee A, McGrane S, et al. Liberation and animation for ventilated ICU patients: the ABCDE bundle for the back-end of critical care. Crit Care 2010;14(3):157.

31. Davidson JE, Harvey MA, Bemis-Dougherty A, et al. Implementation of the pain, agitation, and delirium clinical practice guidelines and promoting patient mobility to prevent post-intensive care syndrome. Crit Care Med 2013;41(9 Suppl 1): S136–45.

32. Davydow DS. Symptoms of depression and anxiety after delirium. Psychosomatics 2009;50(4):309–16.

33. Hopkins RO, Jackson JC. Assessing neurocognitive outcomes after critical illness: are delirium and long-term cognitive impairments related? Curr Opin Crit Care 2006;12(5):388–94.

34. Jackson JC, Pandharipande PP, Girard TD, et al. Depression, post-traumatic stress disorder, and functional disability in survivors of critical illness in the

BRAIN-ICU study: a longitudinal cohort study. Lancet Respir Med 2014;2(5): 369–79.

35. Jackson JC, Morandi A, Girard TD, et al. Functional brain imaging in survivors of critical illness: a prospective feasibility study and exploration of the association between delirium and brain activation patterns. J Crit Care 2015;30(3):653.e1-7.

36. Jackson JC, Mitchell N, Hopkins RO. Cognitive functioning, mental health, and quality of life in ICU survivors: an overview. Psychiatr Clin North Am 2015; 38(1):91–104.

37. Davydow DS, Gifford JM, Desai SV, et al. Posttraumatic stress disorder in general intensive care unit survivors: a systematic review. Gen Hosp Psychiatry 2008; 30(5):421–34.

38. Davydow DS, Katon WJ, Zatzick DF. Psychiatric morbidity and functional impairments in survivors of burns, traumatic injuries, and ICU stays for other critical illnesses: a review of the literature. Int Rev Psychiatry 2009;21(6):531–8.

39. Davydow DS, Zatzick D, Hough CL, et al. A longitudinal investigation of posttraumatic stress and depressive symptoms over the course of the year following medical-surgical intensive care unit admission. Gen Hosp Psychiatry 2013; 35(3):226–32.

40. Wiseman TA, Curtis K, Lam M, et al. Incidence of depression, anxiety and stress following traumatic injury: a longitudinal study. Scand J Trauma Resusc Emerg Med 2015;23:29.

41. Wade DM, Brewin CR, Howell DC, et al. Intrusive memories of hallucinations and delusions in traumatized intensive care patients: an interview study. Br J Health Psychol 2015;20(3):613–31.

42. Girard TD, Kress JP, Fuchs BD, et al. Efficacy and safety of a paired sedation and ventilator weaning protocol for mechanically ventilated patients in intensive care (Awakening and Breathing Controlled trial): a randomised controlled trial. Lancet 2008;371(9607):126–34.

43. Löf L, Berggren L, Ahlström G. Severely ill ICU patients recall of factual events and unreal experiences of hospital admission and ICU stay—3 and 12 months after discharge. Intensive Crit Care Nurs 2006;22(3):154–66.

44. Altman MT, Knauert MP, Pisani MA. Sleep disturbance after hospitalization and critical illness: a systematic review. Ann Am Thorac Soc 2017;14(9):1457–68.

45. American Psychiatric A, American Psychiatric A, Force DSMT. Diagnostic and statistical manual of mental disorders: DSM-5; 2013.

46. Zatzick D, Jurkovich GJ, Rivara FP, et al. A national US study of posttraumatic stress disorder, depression, and work and functional outcomes after hospitalization for traumatic injury. Ann Surg 2008;248(3):429–37.

47. Soberg HL, Finset A, Roise O, et al. The trajectory of physical and mental health from injury to 5 years after multiple trauma: a prospective, longitudinal cohort study. Arch Phys Med Rehabil 2012;93(5):765–74.

48. Falkenberg L, Zeckey C, Mommsen P, et al. Long-term outcome in 324 polytrauma patients: what factors are associated with posttraumatic stress disorder and depressive disorder symptoms? Eur J Med Res 2017;22(1):44.

49. Howlett JR, Stein MB. Prevention of trauma and stressor-related disorders: a review. Neuropsychopharmacology 2016;41(1):357–69.

50. Ozer EJ, Best SR, Lipsey TL, et al. Predictors of posttraumatic stress disorder and symptoms in adults: a meta-analysis. Psychol Bull 2003;129(1):52–73.

51. Brewin CR, Andrews B, Valentine JD. Meta-analysis of risk factors for posttraumatic stress disorder in trauma-exposed adults. J Consult Clin Psychol 2000; 68(5):748–66.

52. Skogstad L, Hem E, Sandvik L, et al. Nurse-led psychological intervention after physical traumas: a randomized controlled trial. J Clin Med Res 2015;7(5): 339–47.

53. Papadakaki M, Ferraro OE, Orsi C, et al. Psychological distress and physical disability in patients sustaining severe injuries in road traffic crashes: results from a one-year cohort study from three European countries. Injury 2017;48(2): 297–306.

54. Davydow DS, Zatzick DF, Rivara FP, et al. Predictors of posttraumatic stress disorder and return to usual major activity in traumatically injured intensive care unit survivors. Gen Hosp Psychiatry 2009;31(5):428–35.

55. Foy DW, Ruzek JI, Glynn SM, et al. Trauma focus group therapy for combat-related PTSD. J Clin Psychol 1997;3(4):59–73.

56. Rothbaum BO, Kearns MC, Reiser E, et al. Early intervention following trauma may mitigate genetic risk for PTSD in civilians: a pilot prospective emergency department study. J Clin Psychiatry 2014;75(12):1380–7.

57. Galatzer-Levy IR, Ankri Y, Freedman S, et al. Early PTSD symptom trajectories: persistence, recovery, and response to treatment: results from the Jerusalem Trauma Outreach and Prevention Study (J-TOPS). PLoS One 2013;8(8):e70084.

58. Lee DJ, Schnitzlein CW, Wolf JP, et al. Psychotherapy versus pharmacotherapy for posttraumatic stress disorder: systemic review and meta-analyses to determine first-line treatments. Depress Anxiety 2016;33(9):792–806.

59. Field TA, Beeson ET, Jones LK. The New ABCs: a practitioner's guide to neuroscience-informed cognitive-behavior therapy. J Ment Health Couns 2015; 37(3):206–20.

60. Mikkelsen ME, Jackson JC, Hopkins RO, et al. Peer support as a novel strategy to mitigate post-intensive care syndrome. AACN Adv Crit Care 2016;27(2):221–9.

61. Davidson L, Chinman M, Sells D, et al. Peer support among adults with serious mental illness: a report from the field. Schizophr Bull 2006;32(3):443–50.

62. Chinman M, George P, Dougherty RH, et al. Peer support services for individuals with serious mental illnesses: assessing the evidence. Psychiatr Serv 2014;65(4): 429–41.

63. Davidson L, Bellamy C, Guy K, et al. Peer support among persons with severe mental illnesses: a review of evidence and experience. World Psychiatry 2012; 11(2):123–8.

64. Boisvert RA, Martin LM, Grosek M, et al. Effectiveness of a peer-support community in addiction recovery: participation as intervention. Occup Ther Int 2008; 15(4):205–20.

65. McPeake J, Quasim T. The role of peer support in ICU rehabilitation. Intensive Crit Care Nurs 2016;37:1–3.

66. Tolley JS, Foroushani PS. What do we know about one-to-one peer support for adults with a burn injury? A scoping review. J Burn Care Res 2014;35(3):233–42.

67. Foy DW, Eriksson CB, Trice GA. Introduction to group interventions for trauma survivors. Group Dyn 2001;5(4):246–51.

68. Whybrow D, Jones N, Greenberg N. Promoting organizational well-being: a comprehensive review of trauma risk management. Occup Med (Lond) 2015; 65(4):331–6.

69. Jain S, McLean C, Adler EP, et al. Peer support and outcome for veterans with posttraumatic stress disorder (PTSD) in a residential rehabilitation program. Community Ment Health J 2016;52(8):1089–92.

70. Roberts NP, Kitchiner NJ, Kenardy J, et al. Early psychological interventions to treat acute traumatic stress symptoms. Cochrane Database Syst Rev 2010;(3):CD007944.

71. Bisson JI, Roberts NP, Andrew M, et al. Psychological therapies for chronic post-traumatic stress disorder (PTSD) in adults. Cochrane Database Syst Rev 2013;(12):CD003388.

72. Ipser JC, Stein DJ. Evidence-based pharmacotherapy of post-traumatic stress disorder (PTSD). Int J Neuropsychopharmacol 2012;15(6):825–40.

73. Bernardy NC, Friedman MJ. Psychopharmacological strategies in the management of posttraumatic stress disorder (PTSD): what have we learned? Curr Psychiatry Rep 2015;17(4):564.

74. Friedman MJ, Bernardy NC. Considering future pharmacotherapy for PTSD. Neurosci Lett 2017;649:181–5.

75. Le QA, Doctor JN, Zoellner LA, et al. Effects of treatment, choice, and preference on health-related quality-of-life outcomes in patients with posttraumatic stress disorder (PTSD). Qual Life Res 2018;27(6):1555–62.

76. Sessa B. MDMA and PTSD treatment: "PTSD: from novel pathophysiology to innovative therapeutics". Neurosci Lett 2017;649:176–80.

77. Morgan M, Lockwood A, Steinke D, et al. Pharmacotherapy regimens among patients with posttraumatic stress disorder and mild traumatic brain injury. Psychiatr Serv 2012;63(2):182–5.

78. Shalev AY, Ankri Y, Israeli-Shalev Y, et al. Prevention of posttraumatic stress disorder by early treatment: results from the Jerusalem Trauma Outreach And Prevention study. Arch Gen Psychiatry 2012;69(2):166–76.

79. Bradford AN, Castillo RC, Carlini AR, et al. The trauma survivors network: Survive. Connect. Rebuild. J Trauma 2011;70(6):1557–60.

80. De Silva M, Maclachlan M, Devane D, et al. Psychosocial interventions for the prevention of disability following traumatic physical injury. Cochrane Database Syst Rev 2009;(4):CD006422.

81. Morandi A, Brummel NE, Ely EW. Sedation, delirium and mechanical ventilation: the 'ABCDE' approach. Curr Opin Crit Care 2011;17(1):43–9.

82. Harvey MA, Davidson JE. Postintensive care syndrome: right care, right now...and later. Crit Care Med 2016;44(2):381–5.

83. Polastri M, Loforte A, Dell'Amore A, et al. Physiotherapy for patients on awake extracorporeal membrane oxygenation: a systematic review. Physiother Res Int 2016;21(4):203–9.

84. Sakr Y, Moreira CL, Rhodes A, et al. The impact of hospital and ICU organizational factors on outcome in critically ill patients: results from the Extended Prevalence of Infection in Intensive Care study. Crit Care Med 2015;43(3):519–26.

85. Bukur M, Habib F, Catino J, et al. Does unit designation matter? A dedicated trauma intensive care unit is associated with lower postinjury complication rates and death after major complication. J Trauma Acute Care Surg 2015;78(5):920–9.

86. Pascual JL, Blank NW, Holena DN, et al. There's no place like home: Boarding surgical ICU patients in other ICUs and the effect of distances from the home unit. J Trauma acute Care Surg 2014;76(4):1096–102.

87. Govindan S, Iwashyna TJ, Watson SR, et al. Issues of survivorship are rarely addressed during intensive care unit stays. Baseline results from a statewide quality improvement collaborative. Ann Am Thorac Soc 2014;11(4):587–91.

88. Eijsbroek H, Howell DCJ, Smith F, et al. Medication issues experienced by patients and carers after discharge from the intensive care unit. J Crit Care 2013; 28(1):46–50.

89. Chaboyer W, Kendall E, Kendall M, et al. Transfer out of intensive care: a qualitative exploration of patient and family perceptions. Aust Crit Care 2005;18(4): 138–45.
90. Davidson JE, Jones C, Bienvenu OJ. Family response to critical illness: postintensive care syndrome-family. Crit Care Med 2012;40(2):618–24.
91. Herridge MS, Tansey CM, Matté A, et al. Functional disability 5 years after acute respiratory distress syndrome. N Engl J Med 2011;364(14):1293–304.
92. Ortego A, Gaieski DF, Fuchs BD, et al. Hospital-based acute care use in survivors of septic shock. Crit Care Med 2015;43(4):729–37.
93. Hopkins RO, Girard TD. Medical and economic implications of cognitive and psychiatric disability of survivorship. Semin Respir Crit Care Med 2012;33(4):348–56.
94. Naylor MD, Brooten DA, Campbell RL, et al. Transitional care of older adults hospitalized with heart failure: a randomized, controlled trial. J Am Geriatr Soc 2004; 52(5):675–84.

The Anesthesiologist's Response to Hurricane Natural Disaster Incidents
Hurricane Harvey

Christopher T. Stephens, MD[a], Jaime Ortiz, MD[b],
Evan G. Pivalizza, MBChB, FFASA[a,*]

KEYWORDS

- Natural disaster • Hurricane Harvey • Anesthesiology department • Emergency plan
- Prehospital role

KEY POINTS

- Hurricane Harvey, Hurricane Irma, and Hurricane Maria caused massive destruction to the United States in 2017.
- Anesthesiologists' responses and commitment to patient care during Hurricane Harvey are highlighted in this article.
- Preparation and planning for hurricanes or other natural disasters are vital, and the American Society of Anesthesiologists has useful resources for guidance.
- Heroism in the anesthesiologist profession is not confined to the hospital and operating room.

INTRODUCTION

In 2017, there were an unfortunate number of civilian mass casualty incidents across the United States, both natural in scope and of human origin. The frequency of natural disasters in the United States is well recognized, and anesthesiologists have been at the forefront of humanitarian efforts in response to natural disasters, specifically including hurricane-related relief, such as that in the 2017 hurricanes.[1] The recent constellation of disasters emphasized the essential role for anesthesiologists in these situations and echoes numerous authorities and the American Society of Anesthesiologists (ASA), who have recognized the pivotal role that anesthesiologists play in mass casualty events.[2]

No authors have any conflict of interest or financial interest to declare. All authors made substantial contribution to the article and approve the final version.
[a] Department of Anesthesiology, University of Texas McGovern Medical School, MSB 5.020, 6431 Fannin Street, Houston, TX 77030, USA; [b] Department of Anesthesiology, Baylor College of Medicine, One Baylor Plaza, MS: BCM 120, Houston, TX 77030, USA
* Corresponding author.
E-mail address: Evan.G.Pivalizza@uth.tmc.edu

Anesthesiology Clin 37 (2019) 151–160
https://doi.org/10.1016/j.anclin.2018.09.005   anesthesiology.theclinics.com

The eastern and southern coasts of the United States remain perennially at risk for hurricane-related natural disasters and, in the fall of 2017, in a historic period, the United States mainland, Caribbean islands, and Puerto Rico suffered the devastating effect of 3 of the costliest hurricanes in history with Hurricane Harvey (number 2 in cost, Texas and Louisiana), Hurricane Maria (number 3 in cost, Puerto Rico), and Hurricane Irma (number 5 in cost, Florida) over a short period (**Fig. 1**). Hurricane Harvey made landfall near Rockport, Texas, as a category 4 storm with 130-mph winds on August 25 and stalled over Southeast Texas with record rainfall amounts, as much as 60 in, in some areas. The storm spent 117 hours over the state, with as many as 90 confirmed deaths.

The impact of hurricane-related destruction of academic training programs has been previously reported, emphasizing collaborative responses by neighboring states for displaced residents and the program itself.[3] The subsequent impact of such natural disasters frequently outlast the visible damage, because physician shortages were reported in survey data for Louisiana after Hurricane Katrina and Hurricane Rita in 2005.[4]

In this brief review, the authors focus on the impact of Hurricane Harvey on Southeast Texas and summarize, from personal experience and expert recommendations, strategies for the preparation, management of clinical operations, and recovery efforts in such dire situations. Continued discussion and emphasis of both the operating room (OR) and nontraditional rescue efforts by anesthesiologists are essential to guide vigilant anticipation and effective clinical care during future storms.

IMPACT OF HURRICANE HARVEY

Houston is no stranger to storm-related damage and flooding: after Tropical Storm Allison, which in June 2001 devastated many health care facilities (including the city's 2 level 1 trauma centers and medical schools at the Texas Medical Center [TMC]), substantial changes and improvements were made in the infrastructure at the TMC (**Fig. 2**). These changes included construction of floodgates, relocation of vital engineering and power supplies from basements prone to flooding, and re-evaluation of

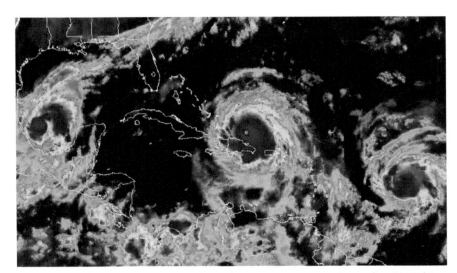

Fig. 1. Image of the 3 simultaneous Atlantic hurricanes in August–September 2017. (*Courtesy of* National Oceanic and Atmospheric Administration, Washington, DC.)

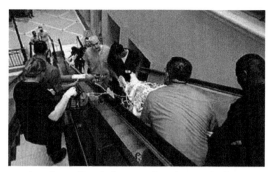

Fig. 2. Patient evacuation from flooded, powerless hospital after Tropical storm Allison, June 2001.

hospital emergency procedures when power failure and flooding necessitate evacuation of the structure (**Fig. 3**). These investments and responses were successful such that hospital function and safety in the TMC remained intact during Hurricane Harvey, even if access to the hospital was challenging (**Fig. 4**). The authors were involved in patient care and rescue efforts, as described later.

One of the authors (JO) was the attending trauma anesthesiologist on call at the affiliate Ben Taub Hospital on the evening of August 26, 2017. Because forecast models predicted stalling of the storm and a slow drift toward the Houston area, with 30 in to 50 in of rain, the hospital hurricane plan had been activated and ride-out teams were in

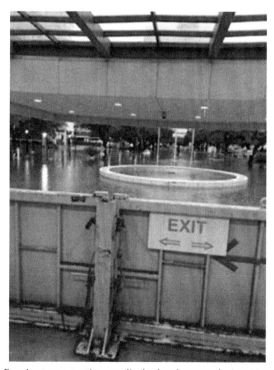

Fig. 3. Successful floodgate protecting medical school access during Hurricane Harvey.

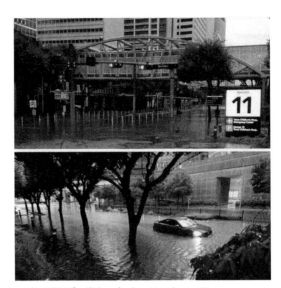

Fig. 4. Flooded access to TMC facilities during Hurricane Harvey.

place for most departments to ensure that critical infrastructure components were uninterrupted during an emergency incident. The ride-out teams remained on campus working to continue essential operations and to facilitate a rapid restoration of critical infrastructure components. Scheduled call teams continued until conditions started to deteriorate with sufficient supplies for ride-out. The street flooding caused water pipes to break in the basement, affecting the kitchen and cafeteria, pharmacy storage, and central supply, necessitating relocation of equipment and use of temporary facilities. The call team was relieved on August 28, and normal operations resumed on August 30.

ROLE OF THE ANESTHESIOLOGIST IN HURRICANE EMERGENCIES

Many departments and programs in potential hurricane affected areas already have policies and procedures in place in anticipation of and during catastrophic natural disaster events. The ASA and the Committee on Trauma and Emergency Preparedness (COTEP) have published cogent guidelines for anesthesiology departments in mass casualty situations and many institutions at flooding risk have adapted or modified these for their own local practice. A stand-alone OR procedure check-list is particularly useful; the ASA manual for department operations is a valuable template for discussion (https://www.asahq.org/resources/resources-from-asa-committees/committee-on-trauma-and-emergency-preparedness/emergency-preparedness).

During Hurricane Harvey, Texas anesthesiologists in flooded areas displayed remarkable resilience in maintaining care for patients, despite devastating personal and family conditions and flooding, with loss of homes, vehicles, and other valuable possessions. Incredible stories have been discovered of colleagues who overcame adversity and continued to provide much-needed medical care, including prolonged in-hospital stays of 60 hours. In the wake of these heroic efforts, potential preparatory and logistical options for anesthesiology departments, guided by the available COTEP recommendations, are reviewed.

Hospital and Facility

As a base of operations in a flooding event, the hospital facility requires pre-event analysis and planning encompassing medical preparedness and uninterrupted continuity of operations. Logistics, such as medical supplies, pharmaceuticals (particularly challenging given the current shortage of multiple anesthetic and life-saving medications), and potentially overlooked considerations for food, lodging, and sanitation space for personnel, patients, and family members are critical. Descriptions and recommendations for response and maintenance of vital hospital supplies and equipment exist, especially when there is displacement and personal risk in nonflooding situations.[5]

During a primary flooding event, such as Hurricane Harvey, there are additional considerations, including potential power failure and contamination of water supply. Holland and colleagues[6] provide practical preparations for OR power failure, and OR personnel should be aware of backup generator procedures and access points in the OR. Storm-related flooding may be exacerbated by structural issues, and damaged pipelines may both exacerbate internal flooding and affect safe water supply. For one of the level 1 trauma centers, hospital evacuation requests were made but, fortunately, not ultimately required.

Usual road transportation to the facility for both supplies and patients may be limited or impossible (**Fig. 5**). In these instances, coordination with local and federal disaster authorities may be necessary to facilitate high-water vehicle or even air transportation options. At a north Houston community level III trauma facility, relief for colleagues arrived in the bed of a truck (**Fig. 6**).

During Hurricane Harvey, the Gulf Coast Regional Blood Center, among other blood centers, had interruption and loss in potential blood donations. Although only a couple of miles from the TMC, due to impassable roadways and bayous, delivery of urgent blood components was made by committed personnel on foot. Although collaboration with the catastrophic medical center of operations is possible, air transportation is often focused on other rescue and delivery priorities. State, regional, and national coordination between blood suppliers allows for import during times of disaster-related shortages. As is usually the case, altruistic local Texas resident donors responded with such overwhelming enthusiasm shortly after resuming operations that supplies were readily available to send, in turn, to Florida and to Puerto Rico later that month.

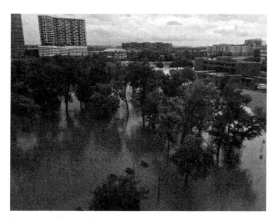

Fig. 5. View from a hospital fourth-floor window—bayou out of its banks, impeding access to hospital.

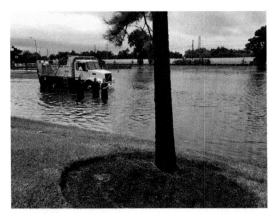

Fig. 6. Delivery of relief anesthesiology team members by high-water rescue vehicle.

Anesthesiology Department

Given the anticipated workforce interruption due to inability to reach the facility or delayed by personal family needs, preparation is necessary to have a viable communication and staffing plan in place. Survey data confirm that anesthesiology faculty and residents do not believe that they receive adequate predisaster event training at their institution. Despite this, it is reassuring that although there are concerns for personal and family welfare, 60% to 80% (depending on the scenario) were willing to respond. The need for training and preparation is emphasized in that a positive correlation is suggested between knowledge of designated responses and psychological comfort with preparation and volunteerism.[7]

Modification of ASA recommendations to a specific flooding event includes attention to the planned chain of command and specific task assignments given the ability of anesthesiologists to use their skills in multiple locations in the hospital, including triage and emergency management. Despite limited patient access due to flooding, scheduled and urgent surgical and procedural needs in all subspecialty areas of large inpatient populations at busy acute care facilities require logistical planning while anticipating coverage of acute trauma victims who can be transported.

Preparation for subspecialty coverage cannot be overemphasized, especially when cardiovascular and neonatal ICU care may be in separate buildings or locations on the medical campus, so representatives and staff from each location must be included in the strategic planning. In a newsworthy event during Hurricane Harvey, a colorectal surgeon at a community level III trauma facility saved a patient's life by performing life-saving neurosurgical decompression of a subdural hemorrhage before the patient could be airlifted later to level I facility later (http://www.tmc.edu/news/2017/10/the-craniotomy-crew/).

Plans for communication should also be made, anticipating power interruptions and cellular network overload, and should include usual e-mail as well as mobile media–based messaging. WhatsApp (https://www.whatsapp.com/) was used by 1 hospital department during Hurricane Harvey.

Staffing and Ride-Out Teams

The ASA template recommends 3 specific anesthesiology teams, although most institutions may adapt to 2. The A (ride-out) team is assigned to facilities during the disaster, typically reporting prior to any travel-related difficulties. Plans to accommodate families are necessary. The B (ramp-up or relief) team assists in prep-aration prior to the event until relieved by the A team. This team also is the one to report back as relief support within 24 hours if possible. C team members provide overall pre-paredness support and are available to return within 24 hours to 48 hours after the disaster to relieve team B.

During Hurricane Harvey, there were numerous heroic efforts of B team relief mem-bers to reach the hospital to relieve colleagues, including imaginative driving routes, walking, wading (they advise looking out for snakes, but nothing can be seen in the muddy water), and bicycle, to take over from colleagues who remained at the hospital. In flooding situations, an added stressor may be the inability of initial ride-out or relief team members to leave the facility if they are unable to safely reach their homes due to impassable roadways.

At one level 1 trauma facility, the anesthesiology call team was prepared to stay for 24 hours to 48 hours with sufficient clothing, food, and personal items. Relief arrived sporadically within the first 24 hours, formally within 48 hours, and OR operations gradually increased as nursing and surgical personnel became available. Reflective of the profession's commitment, there were more anesthesia providers available than necessary, so staffing could be managed by shift until a full schedule resumed. After Hurricane Harvey, 1 department's emergency response plan was carefully re-evaluated, amended, and improved (Nitin Wadhwa, MD, personal communication, 2018).

EXPANDED ANESTHESIOLOGIST ROLES DURING NATURAL DISASTERS

Historically, anesthesiologists have played a crucial role in the initial evaluation and treatment of acutely ill and injured patients, likely arising from the profession's pio-neering efforts within the ICU and emergency departments. One of the authors' most notable colleagues was an early catalyst for the well-established emergency medical services (EMS) system in the United States. Dr Peter Safar, a renowned crit-ical care anesthesiologist and resuscitation scientist, supported the crucial role of an-esthesiologists in cardiac care and resuscitation and a skilled prehospital crew that would expand the specialty to the out-of-hospital setting. This origin of the first para-medic in the United States[8] fit Safar's vision of future anesthesiologist roles and the ability to train prehospital providers. The European model of emergency care has his-torically placed anesthesiologists in prehospital leadership roles, including staffing of ground and air ambulance services to provide advanced life support in addition to search and rescue (SAR) efforts.[9,10]

Unfortunately, there is a paucity of literature describing the role of US anesthesiol-ogists serving in the out-of-hospital setting, and the lack of education and training in disaster medicine is recognized.[7] Although most natural disaster emergency re-sponses require immediate (within 24 hours) deployment, longer-term planning and deployment have been described for international responses.[11] Use of a template of an academic medical center, often combining with affiliated non-for-profit organiza-tions, to provide care in disaster situations has been implemented in numerous insti-tutions. This model may facilitate more focused rapid responses from anesthesiology departments.

Anesthesiologists, especially military trained, are in an ideal position to assist with out-of-hospital rescue efforts. Military-trained anesthesiologists are typically assigned to a base hospital with opportunities to train for expanded prehospital roles, such as flight or field physicians, and members of far forward combat surgical teams. In the civilian arena, anesthesiologists serve as medical directors for EMS systems and are well suited for mass casualty and disaster medicine operations. During Hurricane Harvey relief efforts, 1 of the authors (CS) who is a trauma anesthesiologist, EMS physician, and US Army flight surgeon, was placed on state active duty in Sugar Land, Texas, as the commanding flight surgeon in charge of helicopter SAR operations. Duties included oversight of medical care provided by military medics, primary care for all involved operational flight crews, and serving as an individual operational flight crewmember, performing helicopter rescues in the Port Arthur, Texas, and Beaumont, Texas, areas (**Fig. 7**). The Army National Guard helicopters rescued approximately 40 victims over a 3-day period of SAR missions.

As an anesthesiologist flight surgeon, having the overall medical and critical care knowledge in addition to civilian and military out-of-hospital training is of paramount importance during disaster field operations. Physician training and deployment experience in austere environments support the ability to be primary medical leaders during hurricanes and other natural disasters situations. The authors suggest that anesthesiologists should be motivated to assume leadership roles inside and outside the hospital during mass casualty and disaster events. Anesthesiologists are in a unique position to work independently in critical care situations, provide medical oversight for other medical personnel, and function as overall medical directors for field and hospital triage events.

RECOVERY EFFORTS

In the aftermath of a hurricane, basic humanitarian requirements of housing, sanitation, food, and transportation are primary. Physician anesthesiologists may sustain property damage as with any of the local population, and after Hurricane Harvey, colleagues were significantly affected from the southern (Corpus Christi) to eastern (Beaumont) borders of Texas. Anesthesiology residents and fellows at the 3 Southeast

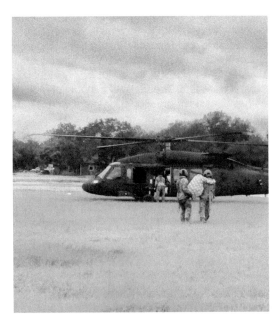

Fig. 7. Army National Guardsmen rescue mission during Operation Harvey Relief; one of the authors (CS) on right.

Texas programs (University of Texas Medical Branch at Galveston, Baylor College of Medicine, and University of Texas McGovern Medical School) were particularly vulnerable, dealing with flooded cars and homes and damaged roofs while continuing training. The Anesthesia Foundation, a related 501-C foundation of the ASA, has had a primary mission of providing low-interest loans to anesthesiology residents for 60 years and had previously provided grants and loans to displaced residents after Hurricane Katrina. The national anesthesiology community was immediately responsive to resident members' needs after Hurricane Harvey (as they subsequently were with Hurricane Irma and Hurricane Maria) and the Anesthesia Foundation immediately distributed financial assistance even before tax-deductible donations began to accumulate. It is heartwarming that these professional organizations are willing to support fledgling members and are a valuable resource option to be recognized for those who may be similarly affected in the future.

SUMMARY

Areas of Texas, Florida, and Puerto Rico were devastated during an active tropical 2017 period. Impact and implications of major flooding and hurricane events, such as Hurricane Harvey, are important for anesthesiology departments and hospital partners to allow for uninterrupted medical and surgical services. Assessment of needs, preparation for staffing, access to the facility, and emergency procedures are necessary prior to anticipated events and benefit from coordination with local, regional, and state emergency services. The ASA and COTEP provide useful standardized templates, which can be used or modified as needed. Stories of sacrificial and committed anesthesiologists during Hurricane Harvey mirror reports from every natural and man-made disaster and emphasize the critical role of the anesthesiologist specialty.

ACKNOWLEDGMENTS

The authors humbly dedicate this brief review to our many friends and colleagues from anesthesiology departments, groups, and practices who suffered personal loss during the 2017 storms and all of those who provided and continue to provide committed patient care during hurricane-related disasters.

REFERENCES

1. Available at: http://anest.wustl.edu/about/news/fehr_describes_work_in_hurricane_ravaged_puerto_rico. Accessed May 19, 2018.
2. Available at: http://www.asahq.org/resources/resources-from-asa-committees/committee-on-trauma-and-emergency-preparedness/emergency-preparedness. Accessed May 19, 2018.
3. Conlay LA, Searle NS, Gitlin MC. Coping with disaster: relocating a residency program. Acad Med 2007;82:763–8.
4. Hutson LR Jr, Vega J, Schubert A. Impact of hurricanes Katrina and Rita on the anesthesiology workforce. Ochsner J 2011;11:29–33.
5. Abeysinghe S, Leppold C, Ozaki A, et al. Disappearing everyday materials: the displacement of medical resources following disaster in Fukushima, Japan. Soc Sci Med 2017;191:117–24.
6. Holland EL, Hoaglan CD, Carlstead MA, et al. How do I prepare for OR power failure? Anesthesia Patient Safety Foundation Newsletter 2016;30. Available at: https://www.apsf.org/article/how-do-i-prepare-for-or-power-failure/.

7. Hayanga HK, Barnett DJ, Shallow NR, et al. Anesthesiologists and disaster medicine: a needs assessment for education and training and reported willingness to respond. Anesth Analg 2017;124:1662–9.
8. Available at: https://www.ems1.com/ems-management/articles/1977832-How-Pittsburghs-Freedom-House-shaped-modern-EMS-systems/. Accessed August 12, 2018.
9. Sunde GA, Heltne JK, Lockey D, et al. Airway management by physician-staffed helicopter emergency medical services – a prospective, multicenter, observational study of 2,327 patients. Scand J Trauma Resusc Emerg Med 2015;23:57.
10. Tobin JM, Lockey DJ. Prehospital resuscitation. Int Anesthesiol Clin 2017;55: 36–49.
11. Jaffer AK, Campo RE, Gaski G, et al. An academic center's delivery of care after the haitian earthquake. Ann Intern Med 2010;153:262–5.

Hospital Planning and Response to an Active Shooter Incident

Preparing for the n = 1

Kevin B. Gerold, DO, JD[a,b,*]

KEYWORDS

- Active shooter • Avoid-deny-defend • Hospital planning
- Emergency medical response

KEY POINTS

- Hospitals are not immune from the changing patterns of violence in the United States, which are increasingly manifest as mass violence and acts of terrorism.
- Active shooter events occurring in health care facilities create a unique set of circumstances that differ from events occurring at other locations (ie, schools and offices).
- Security concerns must be immediately investigated by specialized Threat Assessment Teams to identify, evaluate, and respond in advance to signs of potential acts of violence.
- The response model developed to reduce the loss of life and limit an attacker's further access to potential victims is *Avoid-Deny-Defend*.
- Mass casualty plans intended for acts of violence external to a hospital may not be effective when such acts occur within a health care facility.

INTRODUCTION

Although most health care practitioners live and work in an environment that poses little threat of violence, changing cultural and political norms are giving rise to an increasing incidence of mass violence events. Although the number of these events remain small, the consequences of such attacks are devastating and have lasting effects on the victims and the community. To put the incidence of such attacks in perspective, a US citizen is 6 times more likely to die from hot weather, 12 times more likely to die from accidental suffocation in bed, and 1048 times more likely to die from a car accident than die at the hands of a terrorist or active shooter. For planning and response purposes, such incidents are

Disclosures: None.
[a] Department of Anesthesiology and Critical Care Medicine, Johns Hopkins School of Medicine, Baltimore, MD, USA; [b] National Tactical Officers Association (NTOA), 7150 Campus Drive Suite 215, Colorado Springs, CO 80920, USA
* 1212 Hart Road, Towson, MD 21286.
E-mail address: kgerold@kgerold.com

known as Black Swan events. Described by Nassim Nicholas Taleb[1] in his 2007 book, *The Black Swan*, such events have an extreme impact on those affected. They are statistical outliers, fall outside of daily experiences, but are predictable and explainable after the fact. The challenges facing those planning for such events is that they are rare, extremely difficult to predict and require a prompt adaptation and response following their occurrence.[1] Hospitals are not immune to these attacks. According to the Bureau of Labor Statistics, health care facilities are 4 times more likely to experience violent events than other industries.[2] Between 2000 and 2011, there were approximately 154 hospital-related shootings in the United States. Of those wounded during such events, 45% involved the assailant, 20% were hospital employees, 5% were nurses, and 3% were physicians.[3] Furthermore, in two-thirds of these cases, the assailant had a prior relationship with the institution and at least one of the victims. One such example was the shooting and murder of a surgeon at Brigham and Women's Hospital in Boston, MA, in 2015, at the hands of a patient's son. This escalating incidence of violence, especially in the hospital setting, heralds the need for increasing hospital readiness through health care practitioner education, preparation, and predefined response plans in the event of an attack.

Active shooter events occurring in health care facilities create a unique set of circumstances that differ from shooting events occurring at other locations, such as schools and offices. The preconditioning of health care employees to advocate for patients' well-being and put patients' needs before their own, may impair their judgment to prioritize their own safety in an active shooter or terrorist event. Some situations may warrant a period of abandoning patients out of necessity for a caregiver's safety, as well as the greater good. An uninjured caregiver is able to return and provide help and medical assistance to casualties or resume patient care. Furthermore, it may not be feasible to evacuate bed-bound patients or staff and patients in locations such as operating rooms and/or intensive care units, especially if they are attached to life-support equipment (eg, mechanical ventilators, continuous-renal replacement machines), or patients undergoing surgery or a critical procedure.

Hospitals represent an essential component in our national infrastructure and must be prepared to prevent, respond to, and sustain operations following acts of violence and terrorism. In March 2011, President Barack Obama initiated the Presidential Policy Directive-8, which directed the Department of Homeland Security (DHS) to strengthen US security and resilience against threats posing the greatest risk to the nation's security, such as terrorist acts, cyber-attacks, pandemics, and catastrophic natural disasters. Implementing measures to increase resilience includes preparing hospitals and communities to respond, adapt, and recover from both natural and man-made disasters. Whereas hospitals have well-developed disaster plans to respond to mass casualty events and disasters occurring external to hospital operations, the increasing incidence of violent acts and the potential for acts of terrorism within health care facilities call for the need to create plans for mass casualty events occurring inside the hospital. Such events can occur with visitors and hospital staff as primary targets of violence or as terrorist acts aimed at disrupting hospital operations by creating a large number of casualties within and/or around a hospital facility. During such attacks, a hospital may experience an acute reduction in the ability to maintain normal operations and maintain its usual standards of care. This may arise from the incapacitation of hospital staff and first-responders and the loss of facility infrastructure, as well as the potential for a large number of casualties presenting to the hospital and overwhelming existing resources. Making hospitals more resilient requires instituting changes to detect and deter attacks, mitigate the consequences of an attack (ie, reduce the number of casualties and preserve life), implement strategies permitting an immediate assessment of personnel and resources, and fortify facilities to maintain the continuity of operations. This assessment also must include a determination of a hospital's ongoing ability to provide care to causalities; including plans for the immediate triage of casualties and contingencies for the possible need for transferring the most seriously wounded to other hospitals for further care.

This review is intended to serve as an introduction to active shooter incidents occurring within health care facilities. It provides readers with the foundations for the preparatory and initial response measures to acts of mass violence such as active shooter events and acts of terrorism. For a more in-depth analysis of this topic, readers are referred to comprehensive response guides referenced at the end of this article.[4]

PROFILE OF ACTIVE SHOOTER INCIDENTS

The DHS defines an active shooter as "a person(s) actively engaged in killing or attempting to kill people in a confined and populated area." The DHS notes that, "in most cases, active shooters use firearm(s) and there is no pattern or method to their selection of victims." The New York Police Department (NYPD) further narrows this definition to include only cases involving unintended victims (ie, innocent bystanders and collateral casualties), distinguishing them from premeditated acts targeting a specific victim (**Box 1**). This more limited definition is intended to differentiate active shooter events from gang-related, domestic-setting only, and drive-by shooting events, as well as robberies, attacks not involving firearms, and attacks categorized as hostage-holding incidents.[5,6]

The NYPD reviewed 308 active shooter incidents occurring in the United States between 1966 and 2016. These incidents were associated with at least 930 people killed and 1200 wounded. An analysis of these incidents unsuccessfully identified common profile features among attackers. However, 97% of the attackers were male; the distribution of attacker age was bimodal, with an initial peak of shootings occurring at schools perpetrated by 15-year-olds to 19-year-olds, and a second peak in nonschool facilities by 35-year-olds to 44-year-olds. Ninety-seven percent of attacks were committed by a lone assailant. In addition, assailants are often known or associated with the communities they attack. Active shooter victims know the shooter in either a professional (32%), academic (19%), or familial capacity (6%), but in 34% of cases, the attacker had no prior relationship to the victims. Attacks associated with professional relationships often occurred while the attackers were still employed by the organization at the time of the attack, and many cases resulted from employee disputes.

Although a small number of active shooter attacks are associated with a large number of deaths and receive significant notoriety, they do not accurately reflect the typical event. The overall median number of deaths associated with active shooter incidents is 2, with most attacks resulting in 0 to 5 deaths. The median number of

---

Box 1
Definition of active shooter

Active Shooter: A person or persons actively engaged in killing or attempting to kill people in a confined and populated area, and involving others besides the intended victim, including bystanders.

Adapted from U.S. Department of Homeland Security. Active shooter: how to respond. 2013. Available at: http://www.dhs.gov/publication/active-shooter-how-respond. Accessed July 18, 2018; and The New York City Police Department. Active shooter recommendations and analysis for risk mitigation. 2016th edition. Available at: https://www1.nyc.gov/assets/nypd/downloads/pdf/counterterrorism/active-shooter-analysis2016.pdf. Accessed July 18, 2018.

wounded per incident is 2, and the average is 3.9. The duration of most active shooter incidents is less than 20 minutes, with 50% of cases ending within 5 minutes from when the first shot was fired, or the first person harmed. Attackers ended the violence by leaving the scene in 36% of cases, committing suicide at the scene in 25%, were stopped by police action in 18%, and by bystander action 7% of the time.[7]

PREVENTING ACTIVE SHOOTER EVENTS

Perpetrators often study the methods of prior attackers as they plan, prepare, and in some cases, follow-through and execute an attack. Investigations have identified that perpetrators of mass violence often exhibit suspicious behaviors while preparing for an attack. Some attackers manifest behaviors that raise concerns among coworkers about the potential to commit a violent act. Others may write about their intentions or share their plans and intentions among confidants. To identify potential attackers in advance, hospitals must establish surveillance systems and reporting mechanisms that are aimed at detecting the early signs of potential violent acts. All members of the hospital staff must be encouraged to maintain a situational awareness and report suspicious activities or concerns. Warning signs that should initiate an investigation include behaviors and expressed intentions by visitors, patients, or staff, or inferences that make persons uncomfortable or fearful for their safety or the safety of others. Staff should also be on the lookout for signs of inappropriate surveillance that includes activities that probe existing security measures or test security response protocols (**Box 2**).

When security concerns are identified, they must be immediately and thoroughly investigated by specialized Threat Assessment Teams (TAT). These multidisciplinary teams are trained to rapidly identify, evaluate, and respond to signs of potential acts of violence or terrorism. Centralized reporting to these teams will reduce the possibility of overlooking isolated reports arising from multiple observers. A TAT must have broad authority to investigate all aspects of potential threats, which include the ability to examine social, academic, home, and work situations, as well as assessing a suspect's general state of health. During such investigations, policies and practices must protect persons under investigation against stereotyping and ensure compliance with due process rights and civil liberties afforded under state and federal law. Teams identifying individuals posing a potential or actual threat also must have the authority to refer such persons promptly to the proper authorities or agencies to defuse or prevent danger. Such interventions may include a referral to law enforcement, mandatory counseling, imposed limitations on work conditions, or other actions specific to the circumstances.[8]

IMMEDIATE RESPONSE TO ACTIVE SHOOTER EVENT

The main objectives of the active shooter event response are to prevent or reduce the loss of life and limit an attacker's further access to potential victims (**Table 1**). The

---

Box 2
Warning signs of a pending attack

- Someone expressing vague concerns about potential violent acts among coworkers
- Sharing plans of violence with confidents
- Behaviors or expressed intentions by visitors or staff that make persons uncomfortable
- Inappropriate surveillance
- Efforts to probe existing security measures and security response protocols

Table 1	
Immediate response to active shooter incident	
Accept	Recognize and accept that you are in mortal danger.
Avoid	Leave the area to avoid the attacker.
Deny	If unable to leave, then barricade in a room behind cover. Prepare to defend yourself, if necessary.
Defend	If you are forced to confront the attacker, then fight to disarm and subdue the attacker as a last resort to save yourself and/or others.

Adapted from Advanced Law Enforcement Rapid Response Training (ALERRT) Center at Texas State University. Avoid deny defend. Available at: http://www.avoiddenydefend.org/add.html. Accessed September 11, 2018; with permission.

response model with the greatest impact on achieving these objectives is known as *Avoid-Deny-Defend* (also promoted as *Run-Hide-Fight*). Active shooter events are rare, generally not predictable, and in most instances are over within minutes. When such events occur, persons involved in such acts of violence must first recognize and accept that they are under attack and act immediately to increase their probability of survival and the survival of others. Doing so requires processing the initially incomplete, and often confusing information and acting to overcome the conditioned tendency to deny danger when present. Once persons under attack accept that someone or something is attempting to cause them harm, they must be prepared to act immediately for their safety, as time is critical.[9]

Avoid

The most effective action is to avoid or flee the danger by leaving the area. In a hospital, this may require that health care practitioners charged with caring for patients acknowledge that there is little to nothing that they can do to successfully defend themselves or their patients against an armed attacker intending to do harm. To avoid becoming a casualty, this may require overcoming conditioned thinking to prioritize the safety of patients over their own. Health care practitioners must accept that in circumstances in which patients are unable to self-evacuate or evacuate with minimal assistance, then the best option is often to abandon care. Once the assailant no longer poses an immediate danger, care providers can return and resume patient care and assist with caring for casualties. While moving to safety, it is equally important to call for help and activate the hospital's response plan to notify security personnel and initiate an immediate law enforcement response.

Deny

If escape is not possible, then the next option is for the staff to move to a place that will deny an attacker access to their location. Retreat behind locked doors and get behind cover. If necessary, use nearby equipment and furniture to further barricade against access. Cover is a solid object or barricade capable of stopping rounds fired from a weapon. Cover differs from concealment, which only prevents being viewed by an attacker and affords no ballistic protection. For example, an anesthesia machine or case cart might provide cover and concealment, whereas drywall would provide only concealment. In addition to seeking cover and preparing to defend yourself, remain quiet and turn out the lights, if possible. Attackers denied easy entry to a room will often move on to other areas in search of alternative victims. Denying the attacker access to potential victims provides time for police and security forces to arrive and stop the attacker.

A recent review of defensive procedures resulted in a change that encourages subjects seeking security in a room to position themselves behind cover, close to the door. The prior recommendation was to get as far away from the door as possible. Although this approach was intuitively desirable, in reality it afforded little defense against an armed assailant entering a room. Seeking cover close to the point of entry provides a better defensive position in the event an attacker breeches the door. Once in the room, occupants should also attempt to identify alternative methods of escape, such as a window, and search for items that could be used as weapons should the need arise to defend themselves.[10]

Defend

If efforts to avoid an attacker and retreating to a safe haven are not possible or ineffective, then the only remaining option for survival is to directly confront the attacker. Recognize that confronting an armed attacker directly represents and extreme danger and may require a fight for life. A defense should attempt to overwhelm the attacker aggressively by force and redirect the attacker's weapon. If in a room with others, this can be accomplished with a coordinated group attack against the assailant or by some defenders confronting an attacker in order to provide others an opportunity for escape. In the event you are required to confront an attacker, it is important to appreciate that what you do in such an instance matters and that advance mental preparation for the possible need to confront an attacker can save your life and the life of others. In instances in which potential victims were forced to confront their attacker, they were successful in stopping the attack in 1 in every 6 active shooter events, even though most of those persons were unarmed.

Strategies generally considered unsuccessful in reducing casualties include hiding under desks or behind furniture or "playing dead," as in many instances active shooters have located and killed or seriously wounded such individuals and some instances have returned to shoot the same victims again. When escape or barricade is not possible, the best option for survival is to defend yourself by fighting for your life.

THE LAW ENFORCEMENT AND EMERGENCY MEDICAL RESPONSE

Nearly all police officers now train and rehearse to respond to active shooter events. The objective of first-arriving police officers is to immediately make entry and move to the sound of gunfire in an effort stop the ongoing killing by an attacker. In doing so they will move past injured persons, as any delay in confronting the attacker will result in additional lives lost or serious injuries.

When police arrive, appreciate that they are entering a high-stress situation with many unknowns; officers will be armed and hyper-vigilant. Anyone confronted by police during an active shooter incident should not resist and immediately follow a police officer's instructions. In particular, keep hands open and in plain sight to signal that you do not have a weapon. As the identity of the attacker(s) is often unknown to the police, do not resist if police place you in protective custody, search for weapons, or apply physical restraints. When instructed to do so, exit through the designated safe corridor to a place of safety.

Emergency medical first-responders are also trained to respond to active shooter incidences. Often organized as a Rescue Task Force, these emergency medical responders will accompany or arrive behind police officers and are trained and equipped to perform a rapid triage of casualties, render immediate potentially life-saving care, and evacuate the wounded to areas where they can receive definitive care.

IMMEDIATE AFTERMATH OF AN ACTIVE SHOOTER INCIDENT

Approximately 50% of violent assaults associated with active shooter incidents will end within 5 minutes of the first gunshot or the first person harmed, and more than 70% will end within 15 minutes.[7] In the immediate aftermath, generalized confusion and some panic is expected. Colleagues, friends, and coworkers may be seriously or mortally wounded and require immediate care.

Once the scene is relatively safe, the first medical priority is to reduce further mortality by identifying seriously wounded casualties needing immediate care. Wounds most associated with potentially preventable death if treated immediately are those resulting in massive external arterial hemorrhage and those causing airway obstruction and impaired ventilation. The initial treatment of external arterial hemorrhage is to apply direct pressure and/or apply a commercially available tourniquet, if possible. In anticipation of needing emergency medical supplies, including those for hemorrhage control, government initiatives in collaboration with the American College of Surgeons Committee on Trauma and others, have encouraged making these supplies immediately available by the strategic placement of public access hemorrhage control stations, similar to the deployment of Automatic Electronic Defibrillators in anticipation of a cardiac arrest.[11,12]

THE NEED FOR ADVANCE PLANNING AND REHEARSAL

In the immediate aftermath of an active shooter event or act of terrorism, hospital leaders will need to make critical initial decisions regarding the ability to maintain the continuity of hospital operations. This ability requires advanced preparation and rehearsal in anticipation for such an event. The need to maintain operations following active shooter events and acts of terrorism further distinguish hospital operations from those occurring in other types of facilities, such as schools and offices. Response plans for a continuity of operations must be tailored to the needs of the specific facility. A disaster plan intended to receive casualties following an act of mass violence in the community will not suffice when the same act occurs within the health care facility. Hospital leaders are encouraged to implement measures that increase the resilience of their facility in the event of such an attack.

In preparation for such an event, facilities must develop methods to rapidly determine its ongoing ability to continue essential services with existing working staff and functioning facilities. As a consequence of an attack, key personal may have been wounded or disabled. Sites for normally rendering care, such as the emergency department or operating rooms, may have been the site of the attack. An important initial determination is to determine whether the facility retains the capacity to treat its casualties or if it must transport seriously wounded casualties to nearby trauma centers for definitive care. Hospital planning should also identify alternative treatment areas should the primary treatment areas become incapacitated or overwhelmed. Whereas the emergency room would normally serve as the initial location to receive casualties and initiate care, alternative locations such as the post-anesthesia care unit may serve as an alternative triage and care site, as it is in proximity to anesthesia and damage control surgical services. Preplanning should also define how staff will initially triage casualties and transport the injured to appropriate casualty collection points. Finally, there should be established means to communicate vital information surrounding the event in real time, and rapidly establish clear lines of communications among key hospital personnel, police, and emergency medical service personnel.

SUMMARY

Hospitals are vulnerable to the changing patterns of violence in society that are increasingly manifested as active shooter events and acts of terrorism. Improving the resilience of our key infrastructure facilities requires that hospitals and health care workers participate in all aspects of response plans that would include a means to prevent, detect, mitigate, and continue operations surrounding such attacks. Active shooter events are rare, generally unpredictable, and in most instances, occur over a short period of time (minutes). Such events occurring in a hospital or clinic present unique challenges that differ from those encountered in traditional workplaces, such as offices or schools, and planning and preparation must address those differences. Preventive measures require hospitals to conduct surveillance measures intended to identify and respond to potential attacks. In addition to developing active shooter surveillance and response plans, hospitals must exercise these plans using simulated response drills. In the event of an active shooter attack, hospital personnel must quickly accept that they are in grave danger and immediately implement survival strategies against attackers based on models such as *Avoid-Deny-Defend*. Once that attack has ended, staff must be prepared to care for seriously wounded casualties and assess the facility's ability to maintain routine care operations.

REFERENCES

1. Taleb NN. The black swan: the impact of the highly improbable. New York: Random House; 2007.
2. Workplace violence in healthcare: Understanding the challenge. Occupational Safety and Health Administration, OSHA 3826 - 12/2015. Available at: https://www.osha.gov/Publications/OSHA3826.pdf. Accessed July 15, 2018.
3. Kelen GD, Catlett CL, Kubit JG, et al. Hospital-based shootings in the United States: 2000 to 2011. Ann Emerg Med 2012;60(6):790–8.e1.
4. Active shooter planning and response. Healthcare & Public Health Sector Coordinating Council; 2017. Available at: https://www.calhospitalprepare.org/sites/main/files/file-attachments/as_active-shooter-planning-and-response-in-a-healthcare-setting_1.pdf. Accessed July 15, 2018.
5. Active shooter recommendations and analysis for risk mitigation, 2016 edition. The New York City Police Department. Available at: https://www1.nyc.gov/assets/nypd/downloads/pdf/counterterrorism/active-shooter-analysis2016.pdf. Accessed July 18, 2018.
6. Incorporating active shooter incident planning into health care facility emergency operations plans. U.S. Department of Health and Human Services, Office of the Assistant Secretary for Preparedness and Response, Division of Health System Policy, and Division of Tactical Programs. 2014. Available at: https://www.calhospitalprepare.org/sites/main/files/file-attachments/hc_eop_and_active_shooter.pdf. Accessed July 15, 2018.
7. Mass attacks in public spaces—2017. National Threat Assessment Center, United States Secret Service, Department of Homeland Security; 2018. Available at: https://www.secretservice.gov/forms/USSS_NTAC-Mass_Attacks_in_Public_Spaces-2017.pdf. Accessed July 15, 2018.
8. Cornell D, Allen K. Development, evaluation, and future directions of the Virginia student threat assessment guidelines. J Sch Violence 2011;10(1):88–106.
9. MESH coalition: responding to an active shooter in a healthcare setting. Available at: https://vimeo.com/112455575. Accessed July 15, 2018.

10. Blair JP. The tradeoff: speed vs. safety. The responder, the Newsletter of the ALERRT Center, vol. 4. San Marcos (TX): Texas State University; 2018. No. 7.
11. Bleeding Control.org. American College of Surgeons. Available at: https://www.bleedingcontrol.org/. Accessed July 15, 2018.
12. Civilian Response to Active Shooter Events (CRASE). The Advanced Law Enforcement Rapid Response Training (ALERRT) Center, Texas State University. Available at: https://alerrt.org/course_types/view/98. Accessed July 15, 2018.

Novel Methods for Hemorrhage Control

Resuscitative Endovascular Balloon Occlusion of the Aorta and Emergency Preservation and Resuscitation

Kazuhide Matsushima, MD[a], Bianca Conti, MD[b],
Ravi Chauhan, FRCA, FCAI[b], Kenji Inaba, MD[a],
Richard P. Dutton, MD, MBA[c],*

KEYWORDS

- Resuscitative endovascular occlusion of the aorta
- Noncompressible torso hemorrhage • Emergency perfusion and resuscitation
- Emergency department thoracotomy

KEY POINTS

- Hemorrhage is the leading cause of preventable death after trauma.
- Retrograde endovascular occlusion of the aorta (REBOA) can be used to reduce bleeding and improve proximal perfusion in hemorrhagic shock caused by bleeding below the diaphragm.
- Anesthesiologists should be familiar with the physiology of REBOA and potential complications.
- Rapid deep hypothermic arrest is under investigation as a technique for treatment of cardiac arrest due to traumatic hemorrhage.

INTRODUCTION

Even with recent advances in trauma care, hemorrhage remains the main cause of preventable death after injury.[1] Although active extremity or junctional hemorrhage can be temporarily controlled by either manual compression or application of a tourniquet, immediate surgical or endovascular intervention is required for definitive

The authors deny any potential conflicts of interest.
[a] Division of Acute Care Surgery, LAC+USC Medical Center, 2051 Marengo Street, IPT C5L100, Los Angeles, CA 90033, USA; [b] Division of Trauma Anesthesiology, R Adams Cowley Shock Trauma Center, University of Maryland School of Medicine, 22 South Greene Street, Baltimore, MD 21201, USA; [c] Department of Anesthesiology, Texas A&M School of Medicine, US Anesthesia Partners, 12222 Merit Drive, Dallas, TX 75251, USA
* Corresponding author.
E-mail address: Richard.dutton@usap.com

Anesthesiology Clin 37 (2019) 171–182
https://doi.org/10.1016/j.anclin.2018.09.003
anesthesiology.theclinics.com

control of noncompressible hemorrhage in the thorax, abdomen, or pelvis.[2,3] Delay in control of torso hemorrhage is associated with poor patient outcomes.[4,5]

Aortic occlusion is a surgical technique to minimize ongoing hemorrhage by decreasing distal arterial flow and pressure to injured organs or vessels.[6] In addition, aortic occlusion improves proximal perfusion in the heart and brain. Classically, aortic occlusion is achieved via left-sided thoracotomy and cross-clamping the descending thoracic aorta, a procedure often referred to as *resuscitative thoracotomy (RT)*. Intraoperatively, the aorta can be occluded in the abdomen just below the diaphragm and above the celiac axis (supraceliac control) or below the renal arteries (infrarenal control).

In the past few decades there has been increasing use of endovascular technology in the management of traumatic hemorrhage.[7–9] Resuscitative endovascular balloon occlusion of the aorta (REBOA) is now available at most major trauma centers in the United States, as a temporizing measure for patients with exsanguinating hemorrhage below the diaphragm. Catheter-based aortic occlusion is used at more than 250 hospitals (nearly 150 level 1 trauma centers).[10] It is imperative for anesthesiologists to be familiar with the general principles, indications/contraindications, and technical aspects of resuscitative strategies using REBOA.

For patients already in extremis, REBOA may be insufficient to restore perfusion. Emergency perfusion and resuscitation (EPR), combining the metabolic benefits of deep hypothermia with external support of the circulation, is under investigation as a futuristic approach to salvage in this population.

This article reviews the current literature on REBOA and EPR, with emphasis on how these technologies affect anesthetic management and patient flow through the trauma center.

HISTORICAL DEVELOPMENT OF RESUSCITATIVE ENDOVASCULAR BALLOON OCCLUSION OF THE AORTA

Hughes[11] reported on 3 injured soldiers who underwent balloon occlusion of the aorta in 1954. In the following decades there were only a few small case series describing the use of intra-aortic balloon occlusion for trauma patients.[11–13] A lack of sophisticated devices, a high incidence of major complications, and unclear indications for use were likely factors that prevented trauma surgeons from widespread application of REBOA. In other patient populations, endovascular aortic occlusion was occasionally advocated for patients with ruptured abdominal aortic aneurysms, obstetric hemorrhage, or gastrointestinal bleeding.[14–16] REBOA has been used in the management of severely injured patients in Japan since the early 1990s; between 2004 and 2014, more than 600 REBOA cases were submitted to the Japan Trauma Data Bank. A retrospective study using these data showed the use of REBOA was associated with a significantly higher in-hospital mortality rate compared with a propensity score–matched group of patients.[17] This result might not be applicable in the United States; however, as the median time to index surgery was 97 minutes versus 110 minutes in the REBOA and no REBOA groups, respectively. In the United States, 2 case series from high-volume level 1 trauma centers were published in the early 2010s.[18,19] These studies showed potential benefits of REBOA in patients with noncompressible torso hemorrhage. In 2016, DuBose and colleagues[20] reported the feasibility of REBOA use as an alternative to aortic occlusion via RT in a multicenter prospective observational study (the AORTA [Aortic Occlusion for Resuscitation in Trauma and Acute Care Surgery] trial). Compared with the patients who underwent open aortic occlusion, there was no significant difference in overall mortality (REBOA group 71.7% vs open group 83.8%; $P = .12$). Embolic complications related to REBOA were uncommon (4.3%), and there were no cases of limb ischemia reported. The utility of REBOA was subsequently evaluated in a more selected group of patients (the AORTA2 study).[21] The use of REBOA was significantly associated with improved survival in hypotensive patients who did not require cardiopulmonary resuscitation (CPR) prior to aortic occlusion (REBOA group 44.4% vs RT group 0%; $P = .009$). Several prospective multicenter studies and registries are currently ongoing or scheduled,[22,23] but a randomized clinical trial may be required to determine the appropriate risk/benefit ratio for application of REBOA in trauma.

THE RESUSCITATIVE ENDOVASCULAR BALLOON OCCLUSION OF THE AORTA CATHETER AND PLACEMENT TECHNIQUE

Two types of REBOA catheter are currently used in the United States (**Fig. 1**). The Coda Balloon Catheter (Cook Medical, Bloomington, Indiana) is a polyurethane balloon designed for temporary occlusion of large vessels and/or expansion of vascular prosthesis. A guide wire is required for placement. Recommended arterial sheath sizes are 12F and 14F for 9F and 10F catheters, respectively. Because of the risk of arterial injury and distal limb ischemia related to the use of a large-bore arterial sheath, smaller size REBOA catheters are now available for aortic occlusion[24,25] The ER-REBOA Catheter (Prytime Medical, Boerne, Texas) is a guide wire–free device that can be delivered through a 7F arterial sheath. Recent data suggest that the use of a smaller-bore arterial sheath may decrease the incidence of access related complications.[26] Furthermore, a wireless insertion technique with the ER-REBOA Catheter is associated with reduced time to aortic occlusion once arterial access is obtained.[25]

Details of the insertion technique for REBOA have been described elsewhere.[27] The procedure consists of

1. Obtaining arterial access in the groin via the common femoral artery
2. Measuring the depth of catheter to be advanced using external landmarks
3. Inserting the REBOA catheter with or without a guide wire
4. Confirming the position of the catheter using plain film radiograph, ultrasound, or fluoroscopy
5. Inflating the occlusive balloon while monitoring proximal and distal blood pressure—although this theoretically gives the practitioners information about distal perfusion, in practice the distal blood pressure may be inaccurate due to clotting within the catheter's small diameter.

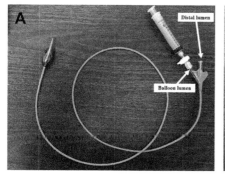 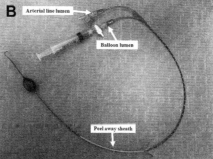

Fig. 1. Catheters used for REBOA. (*A*) Coda balloon catheter. (*B*) ER-REBOA catheter. (*Courtesy of* [*A*] Permission for use granted by Cook Medical, Bloomington, IN; and [*B*] Prytime Medical Inc, Boerne, TX.)

The aortic zone concept has been described for REBOA placement. The thoracic and abdominal aorta is divided into 3 zones: left subclavian artery, approximately celiac trunk (zone 1); celiac trunk, approximately renal artery (zone 2); and renal artery, approximately aortic bifurcation (zone 3). In general, the balloon is positioned and inflated in zone 1 for patients in hemorrhagic shock from intra-abdominal or retroperitoneal hemorrhage, or those with cardiac arrest after trauma. For patients with pelvic, junctional, or proximal lower extremity hemorrhage, balloon inflation in zone 3 may be sufficient. Zone 2 is only a few centimeters in length and there are no practical indications for balloon inflation in this region.

INDICATIONS FOR THE USE OF RESUSCITATIVE ENDOVASCULAR BALLOON OCCLUSION OF THE AORTA

In the civilian trauma setting, the indications for REBOA continue to be a matter of debate. Although there are several case reports about REBOA in trauma, a majority of these reports were from institutions where the use of REBOA is not protocolized. **Table 1** summarizes the potential indications for use of REBOA. A joint statement from the American College of Surgeons Committee on Trauma (ACS-COT) and the American College of Emergency Physicians (ACEP) defines the indications as follows[28]:

1. Traumatic life-threatening hemorrhage below the diaphragm in patients in hemorrhagic shock who are unresponsive or transiently responsive to resuscitation
2. Patients arriving in arrest from injury due to presumed life-threatening hemorrhage below the diaphragm

REBOA should not be used for patients with severe thoracic injuries, in particular those with suspected injury to the heart or aorta. Because aortic occlusion could increase blood flow and pressure to the neck and brain, the use of REBOA is discouraged in patients with severe traumatic brain or neck injuries.[29] **Fig. 2** shows an algorithm to guide the use of REBOA for trauma patients in hemorrhagic shock.

Table 1
Indications and zones for retrograde endovascular balloon occlusion of the aorta placement in trauma

Indications	Zone
Transient or nonresponder (systolic blood pressure <90 mm Hg)	
Blunt trauma	
FAST positive	1
FAST negative, pelvis radiograph positive	3
FAST negative, pelvis radiograph negative	1
Penetrating trauma	
Abdomen, pelvis, or extremity injuries	1
Cardiac arrest	
Blunt trauma	
Cardiac motion on FAST	1
Penetrating trauma	
Abdomen, pelvis, or extremity injuries	1

Abbreviation: FAST, focused assessment with sonography for trauma.

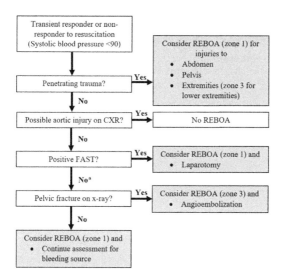

Fig. 2. Algorithm for the use of REBOA in hemorrhagic shock. CXR, chest radiograph; FAST, focused assessment with sonography for trauma. [a] Consider repeat FAST or DPA with high suspicion of intraabdominal hemorrhage.

COMPLICATIONS ASSOCIATED WITH RESUSCITATIVE ENDOVASCULAR BALLOON OCCLUSION OF THE AORTA

Offsetting the potential benefits of REBOA in acute resuscitation are a variety of serious complications (**Fig. 3**).[30,31] Complications may occur at any step of the procedure from arterial access to sheath removal. The list of potential complications in each step is shown in **Box 1**. Some complications are related to patient injury and comorbidities (eg, shock, coagulopathy, and preexisting vascular disease), but serious adverse events due to technical error can be mitigated through provider education and simulation training with the equipment. The ACS-COT has developed a basic training course to teach endovascular techniques, including REBOA to trauma and acute care surgeons (Basic Endovascular Skills for Trauma course).[32] To assure the safety and quality of REBOA at the institution, the ACS-COT and ACEP recently published guidelines for REBOA use and implementation.[28]

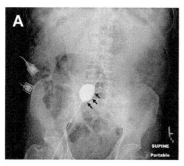
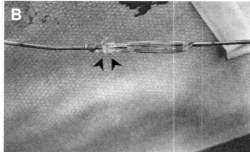

Fig. 3. REBOA-related complications. (*A*) REBOA balloon was inflated and caused rupture of the common iliac artery (*arrows*). (*B*) Overinflation of the balloon resulted in perforation (*arrowheads*).

> **Box 1**
> **List of retrograde endovascular balloon occlusion of the aorta–related complications**
>
> Arterial access and sheath insertion
> - Unable to access or inadvertent venous cannulation
> - Arterial injury
>
> REBOA catheter insertion and positioning
> - Unable to advance catheter
> - Catheter migration
> - Balloon-related injury
>
> Balloon inflation
> - Balloon rupture
> - Arterial injury
>
> Aortic occlusion
> - Organ ischemia (intraabdominal organs and lower extremities)
> - Worsening proximal hemorrhage (brain, face, and neck)
> - Catheter migration
>
> Balloon deflation
> - Reperfusion injury
> - Severe hypotension
>
> Sheath removal
> - Hematoma, pseudoaneurysm
> - Arterial injury
> - Thromboembolism and leg ischemia

PERIOPERATIVE MANAGEMENT OF RESUSCITATIVE ENDOVASCULAR BALLOON OCCLUSION OF THE AORTA

With increasing enthusiasm for the use of REBOA in patients after traumatic injury, anesthesiologists in the operating room will care for these patients more frequently. Close communication among trauma team members is imperative for effective management. A checklist of information and issues for the anesthesiologist is shown in **Box 2**.

REBOA is typically placed in an emergency department or trauma bay, and the patient is brought to the operating room or angiography suite with the REBOA inflated. If the anesthesia team was not present during placement, there should be a systematic sign-out from the trauma surgical team to share information, including

1. Condition of the patient and treatment received in the emergency department
2. Suspected source of ongoing hemorrhage
3. Arterial access (radial and femoral artery) and if REBOA has been performed
4. Balloon zone and occlusion time
5. Balloon position confirmed or not
6. Any complications related to REBOA

Intraoperatively, the anesthesiology team is in charge of monitoring REBOA function while the patient is undergoing definitive hemorrhage control. The team should watch for signs of prolonged ischemia in the abdominal organs (eg, severe metabolic acidosis, hyperlactemia and decreased urine output) and lower extremities. Vascular examination of the lower extremities should be performed preoperatively and periodically throughout the case. Total occlusion time of the aorta should be documented and communication between the anesthesia and surgical teams should take place frequently.

Box 2
Perioperative retrograde endovascular balloon occlusion of the aorta checklist for the anesthesiologist

Preoperative phase

Arterial access
• Site (right/left femoral artery)
• Size of sheath

REBOA catheter
• Type of catheter
• Balloon zone (zone 1 vs zone 3), depth (cm)
• Balloon inflation volume (mL)
• Full versus partial occlusion
• Confirmation image (yes/no)
• Occlusion time (ischemia time)

Suspected bleeding source (abdomen, pelvis)

Any complications related to REBOA insertion

Intraoperative phase

REBOA catheter
• Changes in balloon zone
• Changes in inflation volume (partial?)
• Total occlusion time (zone 1 vs zone 3)

Complications
• Pulse examinations distal to REBOA
• Myocardial ischemia
• Worsening acidosis, urine output
• Change in pupil examination

Hemorrhagic control
• Bleeding source
• Hemostasis obtained (yes/no)

Postoperative plan
• Angiography? ICU?

Postoperative phase

REBOA catheter
• Change in blood pressure after deflation (partial, complete)
• Catheter removed?
• Any complications related to removal

Sheath removal
• Sheath removed (recommended before leaving the operating room or angiography suite)
• Surgical repair of common femoral artery versus direct pressure versus closure devise
• Any complications related to removal
• Pulse examination distal to sheath

The threshold for harm from distal organ ischemia is not clear, so the team should minimize the occlusion time if possible, particularly when the balloon is inflated in zone 1. Options to mitigate ischemia are

1. Partial balloon occlusion (**Fig. 4**)
2. Intermittent deflation and reinflation of REBOA
3. Moving the balloon from zone 1 to zone 3 to control hemorrhage if anatomically feasible[24,31,33]

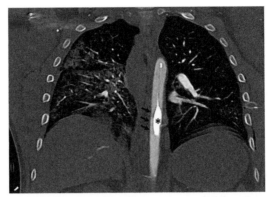

Fig. 4. Partial occlusion of the thoracic aorta (zone 1). Partially inflated REBOA balloon (*asterisk*) and patent distal flow shown on CT (*arrows*).

Once hemorrhage is definitively controlled, the REBOA catheter and arterial sheath should be removed without delay. Open repair of the common femoral artery is not always necessary after removal of a 7F sheath. Any complications related to REBOA, in particular limb ischemia, should be specifically watched for in the ICU, with vascular imaging via duplex ultrasound or CT angiography if indicated.

Next-generation REBOA technology will enable titrated partial aortic obstruction, guided by simultaneous arterial pressure measurement above and below the balloon. This approach will allow for some ongoing distal circulation during the early stages of surgery and resuscitation, in theory reducing the ischemic burden of REBOA and prolonging its safe duration. Although significant research is required to determine how best to apply partial REBOA, its availability is an important addition to the anesthesiologist's armamentarium for treatment of abdominal and pelvic hemorrhage from any cause.

EMERGENCY PRESERVATION AND RESUSCITATION

CPR of patients in cardiac arrest continues to evolve. Although patients experiencing a witnessed cardiac arrest from dysrhythmia or myocardial ischemia have a reasonable chance of survival, outcomes from cardiac arrest due to hemorrhage remain bleak. Hypovolemia due to exsanguinating hemorrhage responds poorly to traditional CPR—little perfusion is achieved in the absence of adequate blood volume—and the limited ischemic tolerance of the brain and heart puts a short time limit on resuscitation efforts. Resuscitation via thoracotomy and open aortic cross-clamping (or REBOA) to maintain cerebral and cardiac perfusion while potentially limiting lethal blood loss can serve as a bridge to definitive surgical control of bleeding. Although this approach can improve outcomes, overall survival of eligible patients remains low.[34,35]

Early basic science research with cardiopulmonary bypass (CPB) and hypothermia suggested that profound hypothermic circulatory arrest could allow for repair of otherwise lethal injuries in a bloodless field, with subsequent restoration of normal cardiac activity; however, the potential risk to neurologic function could not be assessed. Early studies induced a ventricular fibrillation arrest followed by a no-flow state, followed by CPR with low cardiac output, followed by institution of cardiac bypass. Up to 15 minutes of normothermic arrest followed with CPB was associated with survival without neurologic deficit; however, longer durations of arrest led to neurologic compromise.

The addition of profound hypothermia to the treatment (induced with ice water submersion) prior to initiation of CPB prolonged neurologically intact survival time to 90 minutes.[36] Profound hypothermic circulatory arrest of 60 minutes, at a mean arterial pressure of 30 mm Hg to 40 mm Hg, was also survivable.[37]

From these early studies, the concept of emergency preservation and resuscitation (EPR) emerged for use in exsanguinating hemorrhage. Rapid cooling with large volumes of ice-cold saline infused directly through the aorta achieves a brain temperature of 10°C to 15°C within minutes, resulting in cessation of both cardiac and brain activity. After anatomic repair of the site of bleeding, successful resuscitation and warming via CPB are used to restore vital signs. This concept has been tested in large animal models in swine and dogs. After hemorrhage and subsequent cardiac arrest, CPR and conventional resuscitation alone resulted in no return of spontaneous circulation and no survival. The EPR approach increased survival dramatically, with no obvious evidence of neurologic impairment. Adding sustained mild hypothermia (34°C) after return of spontaneous circulation resulted in the best overall survival and neurologic performance scores.[38] For prolonged cardiac arrest of 15 minutes, EPR before the start of reperfusion mitigated deleterious neuronal effects, with higher performance scores and improved outcomes with higher survival rates.[39]

At present, EPR is an investigational method of last resort for patients in cardiac arrest after trauma (EPR-CAT), with enrollment of patients occurring at a small handful of trauma centers.[40] Eligibility criteria include the following:

- Penetrating mechanism of injury
- Signs of life at the scene of injury: palpable pulse, spontaneous respiration, or movement
- Witnessed loss of vital signs lasting less than 5 minutes
- Absence of cardiac tamponade and lack of response to RT and/or REBOA
- No evidence of a nonsurvivable anatomic injury, including severe traumatic brain injury

Initiation of EPR-CAT is an extremely busy time. While 1 anesthesiologist obtains a definitive airway, others place large-bore intravenous access and pack the head in ice. The trauma surgical team opens the chest, cross-clamps the descending thoracic aorta and places an infusion cannula proximal to the cross-clamp. Retrograde infusion of iced saline commences, targeting a core body temperature of 10°C to 15°C achieved within 30 minutes; this may require 80 L to 100 L of infusate in a normal-size adult. The right atrial appendage is identified and opened to allow drainage of infused fluid into the thorax. Cardiac fibrillation and then standstill occur as core temperature drops below 30°C. When temperature drops below 20°C, the aortic cross-clamp is removed to allow cooling to extend to the entire body. The patient is then moved to the operating room and full cardiac bypass is initiated, continuing with asanguineous iced saline.

In the operating room, patients are maintained in circulatory arrest until anatomic injuries are surgically repaired—hopefully quickly. Rewarming commences and blood volume is restored through banked blood, including cryoprecipitate. Transfusion is guided by plain and heparinase thromboelastograms. Transesophageal echocardiography assists in guiding vasopressor requirements and separation from bypass, as the chest is closed. Venoarterial extracorporeal membrane oxygenation may be added as necessary to facilitate separation from bypass.

The EPR-CAT trial is enormously complex, requiring significant investment in equipment, personnel, training, and trauma center readiness. Participating centers must obtain community consent, with appropriate notification and opt-out provisions. The experimental methodology has been validated in large animal models and presented in the scientific literature, but to date there have been no clinical reports on experience in human trauma patients.

SUMMARY

Successful treatment of patients with life-threatening noncompressible torso trauma has traditionally depended on rapid surgery or angiography. New options are emerging to extend the time available to complete resuscitation and anatomic repair. REBOA and EPR are advanced techniques currently under study in major trauma centers and in combat casualty care. Anesthesiologists should be aware of how these approaches work and what patients they may apply to.

REFERENCES

1. Kauvar DS, Lefering R, Wade CE. Impact of hemorrhage on trauma outcome: an overview of epidemiology, clinical presentations, and therapeutic considerations. J Trauma 2006;60:S3–11.
2. Bulger EM, Snyder D, Schoelles K, et al. An evidence-based prehospital guideline for external hemorrhage control: American College of Surgeons Committee on Trauma. Prehosp Emerg Care 2014;18:163–73.
3. Morrison JJ, Rasmussen TE. Noncompressible torso hemorrhage: a review with contemporary definitions and management strategies. Surg Clin North Am 2012;92:843–58.
4. Remick KN, Schwab CW, Smith BP, et al. Defining the optimal time to the operating room may salvage early trauma deaths. J Trauma Acute Care Surg 2014; 76:1251–8.
5. Meizoso JP, Ray JJ, Karcutskie CA 4th, et al. Effect of time to operation on mortality for hypotensive patients with gunshot wounds to the torso: the golden 10 minutes. J Trauma Acute Care Surg 2016;81:685–91.
6. Ledgerwood AM, Kazmers M, Lucas CE. The role of thoracic aortic occlusion for massive hemoperitoneum. J Trauma 1976;16:610–5.
7. Branco BC, DuBose JJ, Zhan LX, et al. Trends and outcomes of endovascular therapy in the management of civilian vascular injuries. J Vasc Surg 2014;60: 1297–307.
8. Gaarder C, Dormagen JB, Eken T, et al. Nonoperative management of splenic injuries: improved results with angioembolization. J Trauma 2006;61:192–8.
9. Costantini TW, Coimbra R, Holcomb JB, et al, AAST Pelvic Fracture Study Group. Current management of hemorrhage from severe pelvic fractures: Results of an American Association for the Surgery of Trauma multi-institutional trial. J Trauma Acute Care Surg 2016;80:717–23.
10. Available at: http://prytimemedical.com. Accessed June 15, 2018.
11. Hughes CW. Use of an intra-aortic balloon catheter tamponade for controlling intra-abdominal hemorrhage in man. Surgery 1954;36:65–8.
12. Low RB, Longmore W, Rubinstein R, et al. Preliminary report on the use of the Percluder occluding aortic balloon in human beings. Ann Emerg Med 1986;15: 1466–9.
13. Gupta BK, Khaneja SC, Flores L, et al. The role of intra-aortic balloon occlusion in penetrating abdominal trauma. J Trauma 1989;29:861–5.
14. Berland TL, Veith FJ, Cayne NS, et al. Technique of supraceliac balloon control of the aorta during endovascular repair of ruptured abdominal aortic aneurysm. J Vasc Surg 2013;57:272–5.

15. Paull JD, Smith J, Williams L, et al. Balloon occlusion of the abdominal aorta during caesarean hysterectomy for placenta percreta. Anaesth Intensive Care 1995; 23:731–4.

16. Shigesato S, Shimizu T, Kittaka T, et al. Intra-aortic balloon occlusion catheter for treating hemorrhagic shock after massive duodenal ulcer bleeding. Am J Emerg Med 2015;33:473.e1-2.

17. Inoue J, Shiraishi A, Yoshiyuki A, et al. Resuscitative endovascular balloon occlusion of the aorta might be dangerous in patients with severe torso trauma: a propensity score analysis. J Trauma Acute Care Surg 2016;80:559–66.

18. Brenner ML, Moore LJ, DuBose JJ, et al. A clinical series of resuscitative endovascular balloon occlusion of the aorta for hemorrhage control and resuscitation. J Trauma Acute Care Surg 2013;75:506–11.

19. Moore LJ, Brenner M, Kozar RA, et al. Implementation of resuscitative endovascular balloon occlusion of the aorta as an alternative to resuscitative thoracotomy for noncompressible truncal hemorrhage. J Trauma Acute Care Surg 2015;79: 523–30.

20. DuBose JJ, Scalea TM, Brenner M, et al, AAST AORTA Study Group. The AAST prospective Aortic Occlusion for Resuscitation in Trauma and Acute Care Surgery (AORTA) registry: Data on contemporary utilization and outcomes of aortic occlusion and resuscitative balloon occlusion of the aorta (REBOA). J Trauma Acute Care Surg 2016;81:409–19.

21. Brenner M, Inaba K, Aiolfi A, et al, AAST AORTA Study Group. Resuscitative endovascular balloon occlusion of the aorta and resuscitative thoracotomy in select patients with hemorrhagic shock: early results from the American Association for the Surgery of Trauma's Aortic Occlusion in Resuscitation for Trauma and Acute Care Surgery Registry. J Am Coll Surg 2018;226:730–40.

22. Sadeghi M, Nilsson KF, Larzon T, et al. The use of aortic balloon occlusion in traumatic shock: first report from the ABO trauma registry. Eur J Trauma Emerg Surg 2018;44(4):491–501.

23. Jansen JO, Pallmann P, MacLennan G, et al, UK-REBOA Trial Investigators. Bayesian clinical trial designs: another option for trauma trials? J Trauma Acute Care Surg 2017;83:736–41.

24. Matsumura Y, Matsumoto J, Kondo H, et al, DIRECT-IABO Investigators. Fewer REBOA complications with smaller devices and partial occlusion: evidence from a multicentre registry in Japan. Emerg Med J 2017;34:793–9.

25. Romagnoli AN, Teeter W, Wasicek P, et al. No wire? No problem: Resuscitative endovascular balloon occlusion of the aorta (REBOA) can be performed effectively and more rapidly with a wire-free device. J Trauma Acute Care Surg 2018;85(5):894–8.

26. Teeter WA, Matsumoto J, Idoguchi K, et al. Smaller introducer sheaths for REBOA may be associated with fewer complications. J Trauma Acute Care Surg 2016;81: 1039–45.

27. Napolitano LM. Resuscitative endovascular balloon occlusion of the aorta: indications, outcomes, and training. Crit Care Clin 2017;33:55–70.

28. Brenner M, Bulger EM, Perina DG, et al. Joint statement from the American College of Surgeons Committee on Trauma (ACS COT) and the American College of Emergency Physicians (ACEP) regarding the clinical use of Resuscitative Endovascular Balloon Occlusion of the Aorta (REBOA). Trauma Surg Acute Care Open 2018;3:e000154.

29. Uchino H, Tamura N, Echigoya R, et al. "REBOA" - is it really safe? A case with massive intracranial hemorrhage possibly due to endovascular balloon occlusion of the aorta (REBOA). Am J Case Rep 2016;17:810–3.

30. Saito N, Matsumoto H, Yagi T, et al. Evaluation of the safety and feasibility of resuscitative endovascular balloon occlusion of the aorta. J Trauma Acute Care Surg 2015;78:897–903.

31. Davidson AJ, Russo RM, Reva VA, et al, BEST Study Group. The pitfalls of resuscitative endovascular balloon occlusion of the aorta: risk factors and mitigation strategies. J Trauma Acute Care Surg 2018;84:192–202.

32. Available at: https://www.facs.org/quality-programs/trauma/education/best. Accessed on June 15, 2018.

33. DuBose JJ. How I do it: Partial resuscitative endovascular balloon occlusion of the aorta (P-REBOA). J Trauma Acute Care Surg 2017;83:197–9.

34. Karmy-Jones R, Jurkovich GJ, Nathens AB, et al. Timing of urgent thoracotomy for hemorrhage after trauma: a multicenter study. Arch Surg 2001;136:513–8.

35. Rhee PM, Acosta J, Bridgeman A, et al. Survival after emergency department thoracotomy: review of published data from the past 25 years. J Am Coll Surg 2000;190:288–98.

36. Safar P, Abramson NS, Angelos M, et al. Emergency cardiopulmonary bypass for resuscitation from prolonged cardiac arrest. Am J Emerg Med 1990;8:55–67.

37. Capone A, Safar P, Radovsky A, et al. Complete recovery after normothermic hemorrhagic shock and profound hypothermic circulatory arrest of 60 minutes in dogs. J Trauma 1996;40:388–95.

38. Wu X, Drabek T, Kochanek PM, et al. Induction of profound hypothermia for emergency preservation and resuscitation allows intact survival after cardiac arrest resulting from prolonged lethal hemorrhage and trauma in dogs. Circulation 2006; 113:1974–82.

39. Janata A, Bayegan K, Weihs W, et al. Emergency preservation and resuscitation improve survival after 15 minutes of normovolemic cardiac arrest in pigs. Crit Care Med 2007;35:2785–91.

40. ClinicalTrials.gov. Emergency preservation and resuscitation (EPR) for cardiac arrest from trauma (EPR-CAT). Available at: http://clinicaltrials.gov/ct2/show/study/NCT01042015. Accessed June 19, 2014.

Future Trends in Trauma Care

Through the Lens of the Wounded How Lessons from the Battlefield May Be Used at Home

Matthew D'Angelo, DNP, CRNA[a],*,
Matthew Welder, DNP, CRNA, FAWM, DiMM[b,1],
Ravi Chauhan, FRCA, FCAI, Dip IMC RCSEd[c], Michel J. Kearns, MD[d]

KEYWORDS

- Military medicine • Operational medicine • Tactical combat casualty care
- Trauma care

KEY POINTS

- The terrorist attacks at the turn of the twenty-first century forever changed the way in which battlefield and operational medicine are delivered. Innovations on the battlefield may serve the civilian population.
- Early lifesaving interventions on the battlefield have led to improved survival of war-related injuries and may prove valuable for civilian health care on the home front.
- Developments in evacuation and early resuscitation en route have been shown critical to modern battlefield care.
- Fresh whole blood and freeze-dried plasma are not new innovations but have found a place on the battlefield and have potential for use stateside.
- Through small interprofessional health care teams and teamwork, operational medicine is successfully providing early damage control resuscitation and surgery far forward reducing the time to intervention.

Disclaimer: The views expressed are those of the authors and do not reflect the official policy or position of the Uniformed Services University of the Health Sciences, the Department of the Navy, the Department of the Defense, or the United States government.
Disclosure: The authors have no disclosures to report.
[a] Nurse Anesthesia Program, Uniformed Services University of the Health Sciences, Daniel K. Inouye Graduate School of Nursing, 4301 Jones Bridge Road, Bethesda, MD 20814, USA; [b] Uniformed Services University of the Health Sciences, Daniel K. Inouye Graduate School of Nursing, 4301 Jones Bridge Road, Bethesda, MD 20814, USA; [c] Royal Centre of Defence Medicine, Mindelsohn Way, Edgbaston, Birmingham B15 2GW, UK; [d] Department of Anesthesiology, Medical Corps, U.S. Navy, Naval Medical Center San Diego, 34800 Bob Wilson Drive, San Diego, CA 92134, USA
[1] Present address: 1538 East Bowfin Court, Key West, FL 33040.
* Corresponding author. 4301 Jones Bridge Road, Bethesda, MD 20814.
E-mail address: Matthew.dangelo@usuhs.edu

Anesthesiology Clin 37 (2019) 183–193
https://doi.org/10.1016/j.anclin.2018.09.008
1932-2275/19/Published by Elsevier Inc.
anesthesiology.theclinics.com

INTRODUCTION: THE EVENT THAT CHANGED EVERYTHING

The terrorist attacks on September 11, 2001, were events that have forever changed the world. The coordinated attacks of Al Qaeda in New York City; Arlington, Virginia; and Shanksville, Pennsylvania, led to the death of 2996 civilians and abruptly thrust America and its allies into war. This single day was the catalyst to the Global War on Terror, Operation Enduring Freedom, Operation Iraqi Freedom, and countless overseas contingency operations where the United States and its coalition partners have been in sustained combat (and counterterrorism) operations, in multiple theaters of war, for approximately 2 decades.

The military response to terrorist organizations has resulted in the deployment of allied combat forces to remote locations around the globe, where they are challenged to operate and employ counterinsurgency and counterterrorism campaigns in extraordinary settings. The present-day, unconventional battlefield has produced a paradigm shift in military strategy moving away from large, unwieldly land forces of wars past to light and expeditionary forces that are dispersed throughout the operational landscape.

The trauma response and medical evacuation systems in the recent combat theaters of Iraq and Afghanistan have rapidly evolved and have eclipsed the capacity of much of the United States, whereby a combat casualty was often evacuated within 30 minutes or less of trauma or traumatic injury. More recently, however, the US military and its allies are increasingly engaged in counterterrorism operations in remote locations across the globe, resulting in greater distances from robust trauma surgical care.

In parallel with its customer, military medicine is evolving to support the new and emerging battlefield. Large fixed medical facilities of bygone eras are being replaced by nimble surgical and resuscitation teams that can move far forward and support operational forces in austere locations. In addition to the special operations community, each branch of service has developed and deployed small surgical and resuscitation teams that provide lifesaving resuscitative and surgical care closer to the point of injury. Given the prolonged medical evacuation times in this global battlefield, the paradigm has shifted from prioritizing movement of the patient to a trauma medical facility to employing resuscitation and damage control surgery near the point of injury.

Although operational military medicine continues to refine its practices to meet the growing demands of its customer, it does so with constraints not experienced in prior conflicts. The shift to smaller tactical footprints requires the development and use of new equipment, treatment modalities, and clinical practice guidelines unique to the austere operational setting. Additionally, operational medical teams are increasingly interdisciplinary and are expected to optimally perform and provide prolonged field care (field care beyond the intended scope of the facility) to patients with limited resources while working collaboratively among the US uniformed services and its allies.

The events of September 11, 2001, will be remembered as a tragedy that forever transformed the lives of every American and countless others throughout the world, and it undeniably changed the approach to care of combat casualties within the military operational medical system. The mission of the military medical system to reduce combat mortality has revitalized research in the delivery of trauma care and point-of-injury combat casualty care, with broad application to the wartime and civilian environments. The result has contributed substantially to a reduction in combat mortality never before seen in previous conflicts. The remainder of this article examines how innovative operational military health care treatment has reduced combat morbidity and mortality through the account of an actual wounded service member, Lance

Corporal Scott Dwyer. Although the service member's name has been changed to protect his privacy, the account is a harrowing description of success. Through the journey of a wounded US marine serving in Iraq, the treatment modalities that contributed to this patient's survival as well as the paradigm shift in operational military medicine are considered and how strategic innovations on the battlefield may have the opportunity to influence how patient care is provided at home and in the future is explored.

BATTLEFIELD TO BEDSIDE: INNOVATIVE TREATMENTS MODALITIES AND A STORY OF SURVIVAL

In May 2006 a US marine was mortally wounded while engaged in combat operations at the Battle of Fallujah in central Iraq. The marine sustained multiple 50-caliber gunshot wounds to the groin, limbs, and head. The Navy corpsman embedded with the unit, who would have been tasked to care for this marine, was immediately killed at the onset of the ambush, leaving no formal medical assets for this squad. The injured marine received initial treatment through buddy aid (care by nonprofessional health care providers) at the point of injury and was quickly transported to a nearby Forward Surgical Team (FST)—a small surgical and resuscitation element with limited resources.

The marine was nearly unrecognizable on admission to the FST. His face and head were soaked in blood and caked in soil. A makeshift tourniquet was in-place on a nearly disarticulated left arm as blood seeped from his pelvis. After critical hours of damage control surgery at the FST, the marine was sufficiently stabilized for helicopter medical evacuation (medevac) to the US Army combat support hospital in Baghdad for further surgical care and critical care support. After additional surgical intervention in Baghdad, the marine was then flown to Landstuhl Regional Medical Center in Germany and ultimately on to the United States only 96 hours after his initial injuries.

In any other war at any other time in history, this marine would have succumbed to his wounds and died. His survival, however, and the survival of countless other combat casualties over the past 18 years can be linked to a series of interrelated actions that include immediate care at the point of injury, rapid access to surgical intervention, and efficient and coordinated critical care evacuation to tertiary medical care facilities back home that provide specialty services and rehabilitative care. Through deliberate battlefield care and strategic health care delivery, retired Marine Lance Corporal (LCpl) Scott Dwyer survived his lethal battlefield injuries, recovered from the wounds, and returned home to move forward in his life. Despite major injuries, LCpl Dwyer has earned both bachelor's and master's degrees and is now a small business owner.

Reducing Preventable Death: Tactical Combat Casualty Care

LCpl Dwyer's harrowing account of survival was no accident and was 20 years in the making through the development, adoption, and implementation of Tactical Combat Casualty Care (TC3). The original TC3 guidelines began as a combined effort of the Naval Special Warfare Command, the Uniformed Services University of the Health Sciences, and US Special Operations Command and were published in 1996.[1,2] TC3 guidelines provided the first prehospital trauma care guidelines for the battlefield that deliberately moved away from civilian prehospital standards and provided numerous evidence-based practices for battlefield trauma care. The distinction between civilian and military care is significant because it represents an early shift in philosophy, where military medicine was no longer a replication of civilian practice but considered unique in the context of war.[1,2]

TC3 is a collection of clinical practice guidelines that are organized into priorities of care based on the tactical environment. TC3 deliberately focuses care on preventable causes of battlefield death and aggressively advocates for the use of tourniquets, hemostatic dressings, and tranexamic acid to minimize hemorrhage and stabilize clotting; needle thoracostomy for suspected pneumothorax; cricothyrotomy for maxillofacial trauma; and the limitation of intravenous fluid to reduce ongoing hemorrhage, hypothermia, acidosis, and coagulopathy.[1]

The special operations community was an early adopter of TC3 guidelines.[3] The widespread adoption of these principles throughout the greater military community, however, would not occur until 2005.[1] Although the full implications of the delay in adoption of TC3 guidelines can never truly be known, data from the prehospital trauma registry provide some semblance of understanding. Prior to the widespread adoption of TC3 guidelines (2003–2006), hemorrhage and mortality for extremity trauma in Iraq and Afghanistan was 7.8%.[4] Despite more than 4 decades of medical advances, the incidence of extremity mortality was nearly identical to that of the Vietnam era.[5] Through the global implementation of TC3 guidelines (2005 and onward) and widespread deployment of tourniquets, battlefield mortality from extremity injuries was drastically reduced to 2.6%.[6]

Reflecting back on May 7, 2006, an essential factor in LCpl Dwyer's survival was immediate treatment and buddy aid. Undeniably, the prompt use of a tourniquet on his upper extremity reduced the rate of exsanguination and provided time for his evacuation and transit to the FST. Although formal, enterprise-wide training of US forces and combat medics in TC3 began in 2005, several combat units began integrating TC3 for all services members (combatants and medics) early in the wars, noting significant reductions in preventable deaths.[7,8] LCpl Dwyer is fortunate to have been in such a unit where his fellow combatants were able to provide care when the medic was incapacitated. The redundancy of lifesaving TC3 skills was a force multiplier in this and countless other examples of combat injury and has saved lives.

Intervention: Casualty Evacuation and Resuscitation

LCpl Dwyer was transported approximately 20 miles from the point of injury to an FST by an armored personnel carrier, commonly referred to as a Bradley Fighting Vehicle. The model of battlefield casualty evacuation is a long-standing tradition that dates back to the Civil War. In this model, patients are evacuated to echelons (roles of care) of escalating care at increasing distances from the battlefield. Typically, injured service members receive TC3 treatment at the point of injury (role 1). Then, based on initial triage and location, casualties are brought to a battalion aid station (no surgical care) or FST (role II) for initial resuscitation and surgical stabilization required. In the more mature theaters of Iraq and Afghanistan, many casualty evacuations bypass the role I and II facilities and are transported directly to the more resource-abundant role III facilities, such as the combat support hospital. Ultimately, patients with complex injuries requiring prolonged rehabilitation are evacuated to fixed facilities (role IV) outside of the theater of operations.

Patient evacuation to increasing roles of care is dependent on the phase of war, the maturity of the theater, and air superiority. The available medevac resources (air vs ground), tactical environment (secure vs hostile), geographic location (austere vs well developed) and weather all influence the flow of casualties to increasing roles of care. Although evacuation technologies have evolved from the horse-drawn ambulances of the Civil War and World War I to the technologically advanced aeromedical evacuation of modern war, the model of patient movement remains nearly the same.[9] Injured patients are triaged and cared for at the site of injury and moved over distances to receive surgical intervention. Although a great majority of prehospital battlefield deaths are due to nonsurvivable injuries, data from the Joint Theater Trauma System suggest that nearly 25% of those who died in Iraq and Afghanistan died of injuries that were potentially survivable had they reached a surgeon.[6] Patient movement is time and distance dependent and, therefore, may conflict with the golden hour.[10]

Bridging the gap between injury, evacuation, and damage control surgery is a theme undergoing intense study in the operational health care community. In addition to the principles described in TC3 military medicine is pioneering prehospital resuscitative strategies by employing en route transfusion of blood products, including the administration of freeze-dried human plasma, and reimagining the role of fresh whole blood (FWB).

Freeze-Dried Human Plasma

Balanced product administration has become a mainstay of modern trauma resuscitation.[11] The administration of equivalent red blood cells (RBCs) to plasma to platelets (1:1:1) has become the standard of care in civilian trauma centers.[11] Unfortunately balanced administration in austere settings is nothing short of challenging. Product availability is 1 barrier; however, even when component therapy is available, logistically managing the supply can be overwhelming. Fresh-frozen plasma (FFP) proves to be one of the most problematic. The main limitation is in its name, frozen. FFP must be thawed before administration and although some higher echelons of care may have thawing technology, it is not universally available. Methods for thawing are not standardized. Unconventional techniques, such as placing a unit between body armor and a provider's body, using radiant heat to increase the rate of liquefaction, are not uncommon. Although the thawing of FFP is a concern in some instances, keeping FFP frozen is another. Operational units are often required to serve far forward with limited power resources. It is extremely difficult to maintain $-15^{\circ}C$ cooling capabilities with limited or no electricity. As such, teams are required to carry large quantities of dry ice or make the decision to thaw FFP before use; however, once thawed, FFP is only good for 5 days in the cooler.

The introduction of freeze-dried plasma (FDP) is a relatively new asset in the US arsenal; however it has been available in Europe since the early 1990s.[12] First introduced in World War II, FDP is not a new technology, but it fell from favor due to the risk of transmission of blood-borne pathogens.[12] FDP has been used by North Atlantic Treaty Organization forces and is carried by selected units in the US Special Operations community.[13] FDP is stored in bottles or in intravenous administration bags and reconstituted with normal saline or sterile water. This formulation allows for ease of carry and negates the requirements for refrigeration and freezing. The clinical efficacy of FDP is evolving, however, based on available evidence; it is now considered functionally interchangeable with liquid plasma.[14] Data from US forces demonstrate that more than 70% of casualties administered FDP with catastrophic life-threatening injuries survived.[15] FDP provides an additional resuscitation tool that has an extended shelf life that is easily carried by the medical team.

Whole Blood

As with FDP, whole blood has a rich history of use on the battlefield, because it was in common use by the US military during the World War I and World War II and has been in use in every major US conflict since. In today's combat environment, FWB is a viable and readily available option to manage patients suffering from hemorrhagic shock in resource-limited environments. It is obtained via walking blood banks, whereby whole blood is taken from US military donors at the time of need and usually transfused immediately to the casualty. It provides physiologically correct concentrations of plasma, RBCs, and platelets (1:1:1). Unlike stored blood, it is not subject to storage lesion, which likely affects functionality RBCs, clotting factors, and platelets and is also a source of platelets in a setting where they are not usually available. FWB requires an ABO type–specific match with the casualty and necessitates collection equipment that includes point-of-care blood typing and screening for blood-borne pathogens. Although the explanation is not entirely clear, evidence to date suggests that casualties presenting in hemorrhagic shock have improved survival when administered FWB compared with those who received component therapy alone.[16] Current military practice guidelines suggest that FWB and activation of the walking blood bank be reserved for patients who are predicted to require a massive transfusion (>10 units RBCs in <24 hours), patients who are in shock or coagulopathy despite ongoing resuscitation, when component therapy resources are insufficient, or in instances where platelets are not available.[17]

The use of type-specific whole blood (FWB) may be limited by the pool of donors who are ABO compatible with the recipients. The challenge of meeting the demand for a balanced (1:1:1) and compatible blood product in the deployed setting may have found its solution in the reemergence of low-titer group O whole blood (LTOWB). Most of the blood transfused by the US military during World War II was group O whole blood. ABO titers were measured during the war and units of blood were labeled either low-titer or high-titer based on whether their isoagglutinin IgM (anti-A/anti-B) titer was less than or greater than 256, respectively. Although widely used during the Korean War and Vietnam War, LTOWB use dropped off significantly in the 1970s, particularly in civilian practice, because a greater emphasis was placed on using component therapy.[18]

Recently, a renewed interest in LTOWB has gained traction in the US military because operations have moved to more and more austere environments further away from reliable sources and resupply of blood products, especially given the goal of a balanced resuscitation. In the spring of 2015, The US Army 75th Ranger Regiment launched the Ranger O Low Titer program, with the goal of identifying group O whole blood donors from within their unit prior to deploying to their area of operation. Donation was voluntary and, once group O donors were identified, in addition to measurement of anti-A/anti-B titer levels, they underwent further screening, including a questionnaire and testing for transfusion-transmitted diseases. Subsequently, other units throughout the US military have successfully adopted similar programs.[19] The 2 common courses of action are to either identify low-titer group O donors for emergency FWB collection downrange or collection of LTOWB premission. LTOWB can be stored for 35 days in citrate phosphate dextrose adenine-1 solution at 1°C to 6°C. LTOWB seems a promising part of the solution to damage control resuscitation in the austere setting and undoubtedly will expand to more widespread use in combat medicine.

Paradigm Shift: Strategic Evolution of Operational Health Care Delivery

LCpl Dwyer's casualty evacuation arrived at the FST emergency room triage area. Although it is unclear the length of LCpl Dwyer's transport time or prehospital interventions, it is known that it was rapid enough to keep him alive. Although FSTs may seem primitive compared with tertiary medical centers in the developed world, they are designed to have similar resuscitation and surgical capabilities as a stateside facility with far greater limited consumable resources.

Although the FST successfully treated LCpl Dwyer, there is a paradigm shift in operational military medicine, with an emerging emphasis on greater access to surgical care for combat forces. Although special operations resuscitative and surgical teams have a long-standing history of supporting unconventional warfare units in austere locations, the paradigm of embedding or strategically positioning surgical, resuscitative, and critical care teams near conventional forces has not been routinely practiced until recently.[10] The complexity of the Afghan theater has challenged traditional medical doctrine. Vast mountain ranges, hostile locations, and an immature and inadequate highway infrastructure present several limitations to timely evacuation of battlefield injuries. To this end, military health care leaders are deploying small surgical, resuscitation, and critical care elements far forward to support the war fighter at or near the objective to reduce the time to surgery.[10] Fortunately for LCpl Dwyer, he was injured within close proximity to surgical intervention. Others, however, are not so fortunate and would likely benefit from forward resuscitative and surgical care. Although there are few case data, Satterly and colleagues[10,20] demonstrate a significant reduction in time to emergency care and surgery for operational forces in Africa when using the US Army Expeditionary Resuscitation Surgical Team (ERST). The ERST is a highly mobile 8-person interdisciplinary health care team that provides austere damage control resuscitation, surgical, and critical care capabilities to operational forces serving in remote locations.[10] Although data are limited, it is more than likely that sister service austere surgical, resuscitation and critical care platforms will have similar impact on operational forces. To this end, further study is required to understand the wide-ranging impact of this emerging model of care and to refine practices to increase operational capabilities.

In addition to the strategic realignment of forward resuscitation and surgical care to reduce combat casualty time to surgery, the operational military health care community has developed forward capabilities to manage ongoing hemorrhage. Although the resuscitative endovascular balloon occlusion of the aorta (REBOA) has become widely used in both the military and civilian settings, emerging innovations like the abdominal aortic junctional tourniquet may be as efficacious as the REBOA and be implemented farther forward by field medics prior to evacuation.[21,22] **Fig. 1** are examples of a junctional tourniquet devices developed by North American Rescue, Greer, SC (https://www.narescue.com). These and similar products may provide lifesaving interventions in the field or prehospital setting. Innovations liked these, along with the capability of providing prolonged field care, may extend the golden hour and provide conduits for survival that were unavailable only a decade ago.

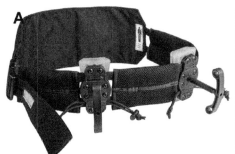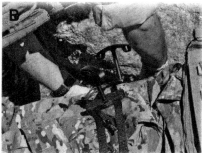

Fig. 1. (*A*) A commonly used junctional tourniquet. Like similar products, this device can be used for pelvic or axillary vascular injuries. (*B*) Once the tourniquet is placed (belt), a targeted compression device can be placed over the suspected site of injury and pressure delivered via a threaded compression handle and pad. (*Courtesy of* North American Rescue, LLC, Greer, SC.)

Although LCpl Dwyer's journey through the echelons of care was exemplary, the US military had air superiority over the theater of operation. Air superiority is a significant consideration and one that cannot be assumed in future conflicts. In the absence of controlled air space or metrological events, operational medical teams may be required to hold injured combat forces for longer periods of time in austere settings with extremely limited resources. As the battlefield has evolved, however, and new geographic challenges are confronted and future conflicts anticipated, air superiority may not be assumed.

DISCUSSION: HOW MOMENTS IN TIME MAY INFLUENCE THE FUTURE OF CIVILIAN TRAUMA CARE

September 11, 2001, was a catalyst for war and spurred rapid changes to operational military health care. LCpl Dwyer's injury and tale of survival serves as an exemplar for operational care; through the result of coordinated efforts a marine survived catastrophic injuries while in a resource-constrained environment more than 6000 miles from home. Although the context of the battlefield may differ from some of the challenges facing trauma care on home front, there may be lessons learned from combat that may benefit the civilian population.

Readying the Population

TC3 saved LCpl Dwyer's life. Without question immediate care at the point of injury reduced the rate of hemorrhage and kept him alive. LCpl Dwyer's initial injuries were not treated by trained medical staff but through buddy aid. Although civilian injury patterns differ[23] from blast and high-velocity projectiles of war, the concept of immediate care remains ever so relevant. TC3 maybe the modern equivalent of Basic Life Support movement of mid-twentieth century and serve to ready the public for mass casualty scenarios where emergency medical services are overwhelmed or en route to the scene. A poignant example of these skills and the types of events that might necessitate buddy aid would have been the 2017 Las Vegas mass shooting incident. Countless bystanders delivered care and transported the injured to local hospitals. Campaigns like Stop the Bleed (https://www.bleedingcontrol.org/) are likely early movements for this type of training in formalized civilian casualty care. Although it can be hoped no one will have to use these skills, training like this may have similar effects on the population as TC3 had on LCpl Dwyer.

Rapid Transport to Care

Although early intervention prolonged LCpl Dwyer's life, there is little doubt that he would have died without rapid access to care. It is fortunate for service members like LCpl Dwyer that they were in close proximity to advanced care. The model for military evacuation has grown dramatically since the onset of the Global War on Terror. The military's commitment to rapid care was highlighted by the implementation of Defense Secretary Robert Gates' golden hour policy. The golden hour policy requires that all injured service members receive evacuation or care within 60 minutes of injury.[24]

Civilian emergency management systems (EMSs) could use the military as an example of coordinated care.[25] Through the military's doctrine of medical evacuation, patients throughout vast planes of distant geography have rapid access to care. Unfortunately, this cannot be said for the US EMS system, where states or municipalities coordinate EMS and transportation to care. The lack of standardization reveals differences in care. A 2017 EMS study demonstrates that response times are nearly double between urban and rural areas.[26]

Component Therapy en Route

The implementation of TC3 has allowed the paradigm to shift in resuscitation. Early implementation of tourniquets has provided a means to initiate resuscitation earlier after injury while minimizing the risk of worsening hemorrhage. Early administration of component therapy and FDP has become commonplace in forward care of wounded service members. Although early blood product administration may not have served LCpl Dwyer due to uncontrolled penetrating pelvic hemorrhage, this practice may have potential implications for civilian trauma care, bringing resuscitation closer to the casualty and restoring critical perfusion to ischemic intolerant tissues. Field-expedient component therapy, like FDP, may serve to prolong the golden hour and provide additional time to move patients to definitive care.

Fresh Whole Blood

The administration of FWB in the operational setting has become a common practice. Constrained resources, remote operations, and access to appropriate storage make FWB a viable option for operational medicine. LCpl Dwyer did not require the administration of FWB the day of his injury because he was the lone surviving casualty and the FST had the resources to dedicate to this 1 marine. This was a rare occurrence. Although FWB is unheard of in civilian practice—until recently—it may be a reasonable option for trauma care in rural communities, where blood products may rarely be used and in short supply or in the presence of mass casualties.

Forward Surgery and Prolonged Field Care

Military medicine has pioneered the concept of forward care near or to the point of injury. The long-established paradigm of patient evacuation has been turned upside down, where the notion of moving patients to care has been reversed to moving medical assets to the injured. Although it is not entirely clear to the authors how this model could complement civilian trauma practice, the authors believe there are lessons to be learned from this evolving paradigm, notably teamwork. Military medical care is dependent on a team. LCpl Dwyer was cared for by a Certified Registered Nurse Anesthetist with the assistance of an anesthesiologist on his arrival to the FST. Through their integrated teamwork with surgical and nursing care, this patient survived his initial injury. The mission and care for LCpl Dwyer took precedent over silos in professional practice. LCpl Dwyer endured dozens of surgeries over the course of his recovery from Iraq to the United States. His care required the integration of all health care specialties. His recovery was grounded in teamwork. Deployed military interprofessional health care teams (MIHTs) are often skeleton crews compared with civilian trauma teams yet they have produced the lowest levels of combat morbidity and mortality in history while serving far from home. MIHTs are composed of individuals who bring unique and individual skills that together result in patient care. Military health care team members rehearse these roles, spend time with one another, and ultimately are able to provide world class care thousands of miles from the United States. Military teamwork could serve as an exemplary model for trauma teams at home.

SUMMARY: SURVIVAL ON THE BATTLEFIELD—SURVIVAL AT HOME

The terrorist attacks of the early twenty-first century have forever changed the United States and its allies and forced trauma care to move quickly in the new millennium. LCpl Dwyer's tale of serving in Iraq, May 2007, is nothing short of horrific. In any other war, at any other time, this marine would have died. Yet LCpl Dwyer's experience, although extraordinary, is a result of deliberate medical strategy, much of which was developed before this young man graduated high school. This marine's survival and the survival of countless other service men and woman are a living acknowledgment of the professionalism and ingenuity of military health care team members and the military health care system. Through innovative point-of-care injury, rapid evacuation and en route care, forward surgical capabilities, battlefield resuscitation, and deliberate teamwork, the military health care enterprise has produced the lowest incidence of combat morbidity and mortality of any war in any point in history. These lessons may serve the civilian community for decades to come.

REFERENCES

1. Butler FK. Two decades of saving lives on the battlefield: tactical combat casualty care turns 20. Mil Med 2017;182(3):e1563–8.
2. Butler FK Jr, Hagmann J, Butler EG. Tactical combat casualty care in special operations. Mil Med 1996;161(Suppl):3–16.
3. Butler F. Tactical combat casualty care: a brief history. Presentation In. 2015. Available at: http://www.naemt.org/docs/default-source/education-documents/tccc/150807-brief-history-of-tccc-v2.pdf?sfvrsn=0. Accessed June 06, 2018.
4. Kelly JF, Ritenour AE, McLaughlin DF, et al. Injury severity and causes of death from Operation Iraqi Freedom and Operation Enduring Freedom: 2003-2004 versus 2006. J Trauma 2008;64(2 Suppl):S21–6 [discussion: S26–7].
5. Maughon JS. An inquiry into the nature of wounds resulting in killed in action in Vietnam. Mil Med 1970;135(1):8–13.
6. Eastridge BJ, Mabry RL, Seguin P, et al. Death on the battlefield (2001-2011): implications for the future of combat casualty care. J Trauma Acute Care Surg 2012; 73(6 Suppl 5):S431–7.
7. Kotwal RS, Montgomery HR, Kotwal BM, et al. Eliminating preventable death on the battlefield. Arch Surg 2011;146(12):1350–8.
8. Tarpey MJ. Tactical combat casualty care in operation Iraqi freedom. US Army Medical Department Journal 2005.
9. Blaisdell FW. Medical advances during the Civil War. Arch Surg 1988;123(9): 1045–50.
10. D'Angelo M, Losch J, Smith B, et al. Expeditionary resuscitation surgical team: the US Army's Initiative to Provide Damage Control Resuscitation and Surgery to Forces in Austere Settings. J Spec Oper Med 2017;17(4):76–9.
11. Cantle PM, Cotton BA. Balanced resuscitation in trauma management. Surg Clin North Am 2017;97(5):999–1014.
12. Pusateri AE, Given MB, Schreiber MA, et al. Dried plasma: state of the science and recent developments. Transfusion 2016;56(Suppl 2):S128–39.
13. Martinaud C, Ausset S, Deshayes AV, et al. Use of freeze-dried plasma in French intensive care unit in Afghanistan. J Trauma 2011;71(6):1761–4 [discussion: 1764–5].
14. Huebner BR, Moore EE, Moore HB, et al. Freeze-dried plasma enhances clot formation and inhibits fibrinolysis in the presence of tissue plasminogen activator similar to pooled liquid plasma. Transfusion 2017;57(8):2007–15.
15. Soares JM. Saving lives with freeze-dried plasma. 2017. Available at: https://www.army.mil/article/197409/saving_lives_with_freeze_dried_plasma. Accessed June 6, 2018.
16. Spinella PC, Perkins JG, Grathwohl KW, et al. Warm fresh whole blood is independently associated with improved survival for patients with combat-related traumatic injuries. J Trauma 2009;66(4 Suppl):S69–76.

17. Whole Blood Transfusion (CPG ID: 21). In. Joint trauma system clinical practice guideline: joint trauma system. 2018.
18. Strandenes G, Berseus O, Cap AP, et al. Low titer group O whole blood in emergency situations. Shock 2014;41(Suppl 1):70–5.
19. Director ABP. Advances in the use of whole blood in combat trauma resuscitation defense health board. 2016. Available at: https://docplayer.net/30983053-Advances-in-the-use-of-whole-blood-in-combat-trauma-resuscitation-defense-health-board.html. Accessed July 1, 2018.
20. Satterly S, McGrane O, Frawley T, et al. Special operations force risk reduction: integration of expeditionary surgical and resuscitation teams. J Spec Oper Med 2018;18(2):49–52.
21. Rall J, Cox JM, Maddry J. The use of the abdominal aortic and junctional tourniquet during cardiopulmonary resuscitation following traumatic cardiac arrest in swine. Mil Med 2017;182(9–10):e2001–5.
22. Rall JM, Redman TT, Ross EM, et al. Comparison of zone 3 resuscitative endovascular balloon occlusion of the aorta and the abdominal aortic and junctional tourniquet in a model of junctional hemorrhage in swine. J Surg Res 2018;226:31–9.
23. Singh AK, Ditkofsky NG, York JD, et al. Blast injuries: from improvised explosive device blasts to the Boston marathon bombing. Radiographics 2016;36(1):295–307.
24. Howard JT, Kotwal RS, Santos-Lazada AR, et al. Reexamination of a battlefield trauma golden hour policy. J Trauma Acute Care Surg 2018;84(1):11–8.
25. Bailey JA, Morrison JJ, Rasmussen TE. Military trauma system in Afghanistan: lessons for civil systems? Curr Opin Crit Care 2013;19(6):569–77.
26. Mell HK, Mumma SN, Hiestand B, et al. Emergency medical services response times in rural, suburban, and urban areas. JAMA Surg 2017;152(10):983–4.

Moving?

Make sure your subscription moves with you!

To notify us of your new address, find your **Clinics Account Number** (located on your mailing label above your name), and contact customer service at:

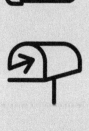

Email: journalscustomerservice-usa@elsevier.com

800-654-2452 (subscribers in the U.S. & Canada)
314-447-8871 (subscribers outside of the U.S. & Canada)

Fax number: 314-447-8029

Elsevier Health Sciences Division
Subscription Customer Service
3251 Riverport Lane
Maryland Heights, MO 63043

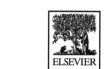

Printed and bound by CPI Group (UK) Ltd, Croydon, CR0 4YY

08/05/2025

01864745-0002